# Embracing Gua Sha

## Traditional Techniques for Modern Living

Mei Lin Zhang

Xspurts.com

**A New Zealand Designed Product**

# Other Versions Available

Why limit yourself to just one format?

This book is now available in physical, digital, and audiobook options.

Choose the way you love to read and dive into the story today. You won't regret it!

**Digital ISBN:** 9781776968251
**Physical ISBN:** 9781776968244
**Audio ISBN:**

To obtain a different format of this book at a discounted price, please get in touch with us at:

http://isbn.xspurts.com/

# Contents

# Have Questions / Comments?

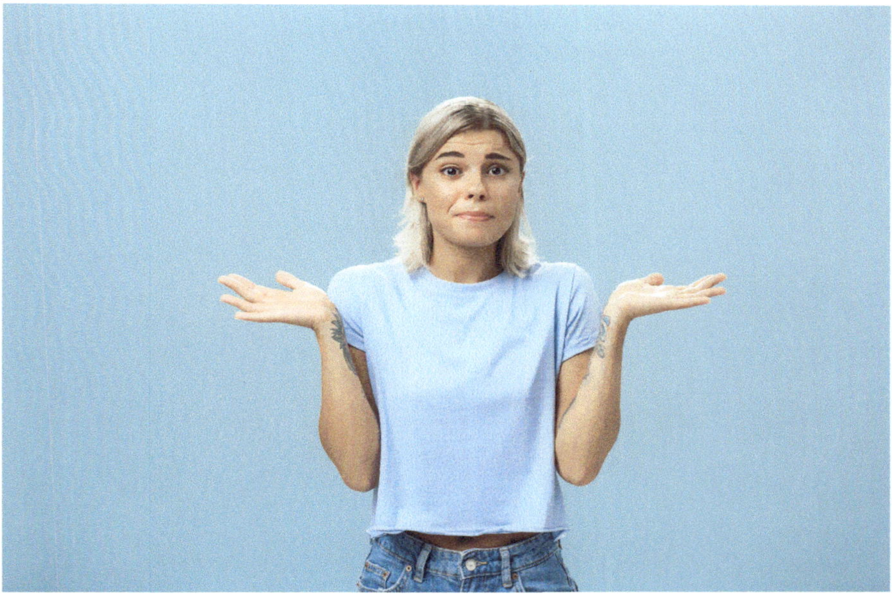

This book was designed to cover as much information as possible, but I know I have probably missed something, or some new amazing discovery has just come out.

If you notice something missing or have a question that I failed to answer, please get in touch and let me know. If I can, I will email you an answer and also update the book so others can also benefit from it.

Thanks For Being Awesome :)

**Submit Your Questions / Comments At:**

**https://questions.xspurts.com**

# Get Free Stuff

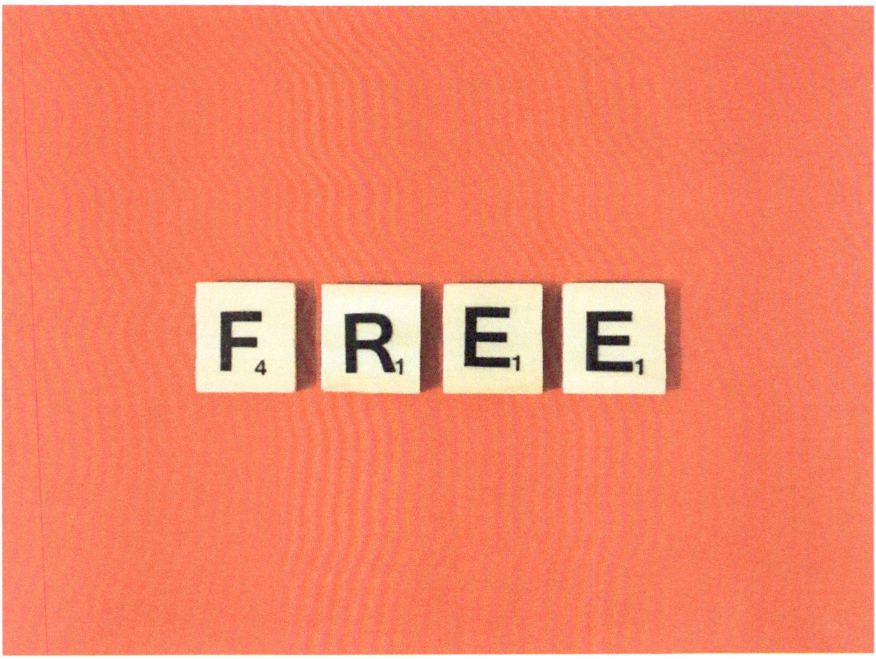


We love writing and have produced a huge number of books.

For being one of our amazing readers, we would love to offer you more books we have created, 100% free.

To claim this limited time special offer, simply go to the site below and enter your name and email address.

You will then receive loads (as we love our readers so much :) of our great books, content and audio direct to your email account, 100% free!

**Get Loads of FREE Stuff at:**

**https://free.xspurts.com**

Chapter One

# Introduction to Gua Sha

Gua Sha is a traditional Chinese medicine technique that involves using a smooth-edged tool to scrape the skin in a firm and repetitive manner. While it has been used for centuries in China and other parts of Asia, it is only now gaining popularity in the Western world as a holistic health practice. Below we will explore the history, benefits, and techniques of Gua Sha.

The History of Gua Sha

Gua Sha has been used for thousands of years in China as a way to treat a variety of ailments. In Chinese, "Gua" means to scrape, and "Sha" refers to the redness that appears on the skin after scraping. The technique was traditionally used to treat conditions such as fever, muscle pain, and respiratory issues. It was also used as a way to prevent and treat common illnesses such as the flu.

In traditional Chinese medicine, it is believed that Gua Sha works by promoting the flow of Qi (pronounced "chee"), which is the vital life force energy that flows through the body. By stimulating the flow of Qi, Gua Sha is thought to help improve circulation, reduce inflammation, and promote healing.

Benefits of Gua Sha

Today, Gua Sha is used for a variety of health and beauty benefits. One of the most common uses is for pain relief. Many people use Gua Sha to alleviate muscle and joint pain, especially in the neck, shoulders, and back. It has also been used to treat headaches and migraines.

In addition to pain relief, Gua Sha is believed to have a variety of other health benefits. It is thought to help boost the immune system, improve circulation, and reduce inflammation. Some practitioners also believe that Gua Sha can help improve digestion, promote lymphatic drainage, and even help with skin health.

One of the most popular uses of Gua Sha today is for facial rejuvenation. Gua Sha is believed to help improve blood flow and lymphatic drainage in the face, which can help reduce puffiness, dark circles, and fine lines. It is also believed to help promote a healthy glow and improve skin tone.

Techniques of Gua Sha

Gua Sha can be performed on many parts of the body, including the face, neck, back, arms, and legs. The technique involves using a smooth-edged tool, such as a ceramic spoon or a jade stone, to scrape the skin in a firm and repetitive manner. The tool is typically held at a 45-degree angle to the skin and moved in a downward and outward motion.

When performing Gua Sha, it is important to use a light touch and avoid pressing too hard, as this can cause bruising and damage to the skin. It is also important to use a lubricant, such as oil or lotion, to help the tool glide smoothly over the skin.

For facial Gua Sha, the technique is typically performed in a specific sequence, starting at the neck and working upwards towards the forehead. The practitioner will typically use light pressure around the eyes and other sensitive areas.

## History and origins

The history and origins of Gua Sha can be traced back to ancient China, where it was used as a way to treat a variety of ailments. In Chinese medicine, it is believed that the body is composed of Qi (pronounced "chee"), which is the vital energy that flows through the body. Gua Sha is believed to work by promoting the flow of Qi, which can help improve circulation, reduce inflammation, and promote healing.

The exact origins of Gua Sha are not well-documented, but it is believed to have been used in China for thousands of years. In fact, the first written documentation of Gua Sha can be found in the Ming Dynasty (1368-1644) medical text, "Ben Cao Gang Mu," which describes the technique as a way to treat a variety of illnesses.

Gua Sha was traditionally used as a way to treat conditions such as fever, muscle pain, and respiratory issues. It was also used as a way to prevent and treat common illnesses such as the flu. In Chinese medicine, it was believed that Gua Sha worked by promoting the flow of Qi and blood, which could help to remove blockages and restore balance to the body.

Over time, Gua Sha became an important part of Chinese medicine and was used by practitioners throughout China and other parts of Asia. It was often used in conjunction with other traditional Chinese medicine techniques, such as acupuncture and cupping, to help improve overall health and well-being.

In recent years, Gua Sha has gained popularity in the Western world as a holistic health practice. While it was once relatively unknown outside of Asia, it is now being embraced by people around the world who are looking for natural and effective ways to improve their health.

Today, Gua Sha is used for a variety of health and beauty benefits. It is commonly used for pain relief, especially in the neck, shoulders, and back.

It is also used to treat headaches and migraines, as well as respiratory issues such as asthma and bronchitis.

In addition to pain relief, Gua Sha is believed to have a variety of other health benefits. It is thought to help boost the immune system, improve circulation, and reduce inflammation. Some practitioners also believe that Gua Sha can help improve digestion, promote lymphatic drainage, and even help with skin health.

One of the most popular uses of Gua Sha today is for facial rejuvenation. Gua Sha is believed to help improve blood flow and lymphatic drainage in the face, which can help reduce puffiness, dark circles, and fine lines. It is also believed to help promote a healthy glow and improve skin tone.

Gua Sha techniques can vary depending on the specific condition being treated and the practitioner performing the technique. However, the basic technique involves using a smooth-edged tool, such as a ceramic spoon or a jade stone, to scrape the skin in a firm and repetitive manner. The tool is typically held at a 45-degree angle to the skin and moved in a downward and outward motion.

When performing Gua Sha, it is important to use a light touch and avoid pressing too hard, as this can cause bruising and damage to the skin. It is also important to use a lubricant, such as oil or lotion, to help the tool glide smoothly over the skin.

## Principles and benefits

Gua Sha is a traditional Chinese medicine technique that involves using a smooth-edged tool to scrape the skin in a firm and repetitive manner. While it has been used for centuries in China and other parts of Asia, it is only now gaining popularity in the Western world as a holistic health practice. Below we will explore the principles and benefits of Gua Sha.

Principles of Gua Sha

Gua Sha is based on the principles of traditional Chinese medicine, which views the body as a system of interconnected parts that must be in balance in order for optimal health. According to this theory, the flow of Qi (pronounced "chee"), or vital energy, must be smooth and unimpeded in order for the body to function properly.

In traditional Chinese medicine, it is believed that illness and pain result from blockages or disruptions in the flow of Qi. Gua Sha is thought to work by promoting the flow of Qi, which can help to remove these blockages and restore balance to the body.

The technique is typically performed using a smooth-edged tool, such as a ceramic spoon or a jade stone. The tool is held at a 45-degree angle to the skin and moved in a downward and outward motion, often in a specific sequence that corresponds to the meridians, or energy channels, of the body.

Benefits of Gua Sha

Gua Sha is believed to have a variety of health benefits. One of the most common uses is for pain relief. Many people use Gua Sha to alleviate muscle and joint pain, especially in the neck, shoulders, and back. It has also been used to treat headaches and migraines.

In addition to pain relief, Gua Sha is thought to have a variety of other health benefits. It is believed to help boost the immune system, improve circulation, and reduce inflammation. Some practitioners also believe that Gua Sha can help improve digestion, promote lymphatic drainage, and even help with skin health.

One of the most popular uses of Gua Sha today is for facial rejuvenation. Gua Sha is believed to help improve blood flow and lymphatic drainage in the face, which can help reduce puffiness, dark circles, and fine lines. It is also believed to help promote a healthy glow and improve skin tone.

Gua Sha is also used as a way to promote overall health and well-being. Many people use it as a form of self-care or as a way to reduce stress and anxiety. Some practitioners even believe that Gua Sha can help to prevent illness and disease by promoting a healthy balance of Qi in the body.

It is important to note that while Gua Sha has many potential benefits, it is not a substitute for medical treatment. It is always important to consult with a healthcare provider before using any new health practices or supplements.

Techniques of Gua Sha

Gua Sha can be performed on many parts of the body, including the face, neck, back, arms, and legs. The technique involves using a smooth-edged tool to scrape the skin in a firm and repetitive manner. The tool is typically held at a 45-degree angle to the skin and moved in a downward and outward motion.

When performing Gua Sha, it is important to use a light touch and avoid pressing too hard, as this can cause bruising and damage to the skin. It is also important to use a lubricant, such as oil or lotion, to help the tool glide smoothly over the skin.

For facial Gua Sha, the technique is typically performed in a specific sequence, starting at the neck and working upwards towards the forehead. The practitioner will typically use light pressure around the eyes and other sensitive areas.

Chapter Two

# Gua Sha Tools and Materials

Gua Sha is a traditional Chinese medicine technique that involves using a smooth-edged tool to scrape the skin in a firm and repetitive manner. The tool used for Gua Sha is an important aspect of the technique, as it can affect the effectiveness and safety of the treatment. Below we will explore the different types of Gua Sha tools and materials used in the practice.

Types of Gua Sha Tools

There are several different types of Gua Sha tools that can be used in the practice. The most commonly used tools include:

Ceramic Spoon - A ceramic spoon is a smooth, flat tool that is shaped like a spoon. It is typically used for facial Gua Sha, as it is gentle and can easily contour to the curves of the face.

Jade Stone - A jade stone is a smooth, flat tool that is made from natural jade. It is often used for facial Gua Sha, as it is cool to the touch and can help reduce inflammation and puffiness in the face.

Metal Tool - A metal tool is a smooth, flat tool that is made from metal, such as stainless steel or brass. It is often used for larger areas of the body, such as the back or legs.

Buffalo Horn - A buffalo horn tool is a smooth, curved tool that is made from the horn of a water buffalo. It is often used for facial Gua Sha, as it is gentle and can easily contour to the curves of the face.

## Materials Used in Gua Sha

In addition to the tools used for Gua Sha, there are several materials that are commonly used in the practice. These materials can help to enhance the effectiveness and safety of the treatment. Some of the most commonly used materials include:

Lubricant - A lubricant, such as oil or lotion, is used to help the Gua Sha tool glide smoothly over the skin. This can help to prevent bruising and damage to the skin.

Cleaning Solution - A cleaning solution, such as rubbing alcohol, is used to disinfect the Gua Sha tool before and after use. This can help to prevent the spread of bacteria and other pathogens.

Towel or Cloth - A towel or cloth is used to wipe away any excess lubricant or debris from the skin after the Gua Sha treatment.

Disposable Gloves - Disposable gloves are often used by practitioners to help prevent the spread of bacteria and other pathogens during the Gua Sha treatment.

## Choosing the Right Gua Sha Tool and Materials

When choosing a Gua Sha tool and materials, it is important to consider the specific needs of the individual and the condition being treated. For example, a ceramic spoon may be the best choice for facial Gua Sha, while a metal tool may be better suited for larger areas of the body.

It is also important to choose high-quality tools and materials that are designed specifically for Gua Sha. Low-quality tools can be dangerous and may not provide the desired results.

In addition, it is important to follow proper hygiene and safety protocols when using Gua Sha tools and materials. This includes disinfecting the tools before and after use, using disposable gloves to prevent the spread of bacteria, and avoiding pressing too hard on the skin to prevent bruising and damage.

## Types of tools

Gua Sha is a traditional Chinese medicine technique that involves using a smooth-edged tool to scrape the skin in a firm and repetitive manner. The type of Gua Sha tool used in the practice can vary depending on the specific condition being treated and the practitioner performing the technique. Below we will explore the different types of Gua Sha tools used in the practice.

Ceramic Spoon

A ceramic spoon is a smooth, flat tool that is shaped like a spoon. It is typically used for facial Gua Sha, as it is gentle and can easily contour to the curves of the face. The smooth surface of the spoon can help to reduce friction on the skin, which can prevent bruising and damage. Some ceramic spoons also have a textured surface that can be used for deeper massage.

Jade Stone

A jade stone is a smooth, flat tool that is made from natural jade. It is often used for facial Gua Sha, as it is cool to the touch and can help reduce inflammation and puffiness in the face. The smooth surface of the jade stone can help to reduce friction on the skin, which can prevent bruising and damage. Some jade stones also have a textured surface that can be used for deeper massage.

Metal Tool

A metal tool is a smooth, flat tool that is made from metal, such as stainless steel or brass. It is often used for larger areas of the body, such as the back or legs. The smooth surface of the metal tool can help to reduce friction on the skin, which can prevent bruising and damage. Some metal tools also have a textured surface that can be used for deeper massage.

Buffalo Horn

A buffalo horn tool is a smooth, curved tool that is made from the horn of a water buffalo. It is often used for facial Gua Sha, as it is gentle and can easily contour to the curves of the face. The smooth surface of the buffalo horn can help to reduce friction on the skin, which can prevent bruising and damage. Some buffalo horn tools also have a textured surface that can be used for deeper massage.

Other Materials

In addition to the tools listed above, other materials may be used in Gua Sha practice to enhance the effectiveness and safety of the treatment. These materials can include lubricants, cleaning solutions, towels or cloths, and disposable gloves.

Lubricants

A lubricant, such as oil or lotion, is used to help the Gua Sha tool glide smoothly over the skin. This can help to prevent bruising and damage to the skin. Lubricants can also help to nourish and hydrate the skin, making it more pliable and receptive to the treatment.

Cleaning Solutions

A cleaning solution, such as rubbing alcohol, is used to disinfect the Gua Sha tool before and after use. This can help to prevent the spread of bacteria and other pathogens. Cleaning solutions can also help to remove any oils or debris from the tool, making it more effective and safe to use.

Towels or Cloths

A towel or cloth is used to wipe away any excess lubricant or debris from the skin after the Gua Sha treatment. This can help to prevent clogging of the pores and can leave the skin feeling refreshed and clean.

Disposable Gloves

Disposable gloves are often used by practitioners to help prevent the spread of bacteria and other pathogens during the Gua Sha treatment. Gloves can also help to prevent skin irritation or allergic reactions in sensitive individuals.

## Lubricants and oils

Gua Sha is a traditional Chinese medicine technique that involves using a smooth-edged tool to scrape the skin in a firm and repetitive manner. Lubricants and oils are often used in Gua Sha practice to help the tool glide smoothly over the skin and prevent bruising or damage. Below we will explore the different types of lubricants and oils used in Gua Sha practice.

Types of Lubricants and Oils

There are several different types of lubricants and oils that can be used in Gua Sha practice. Some of the most commonly used lubricants and oils include:

Coconut Oil - Coconut oil is a natural lubricant that is commonly used in Gua Sha practice. It has moisturizing and nourishing properties that can help to hydrate the skin and reduce friction during the treatment. Coconut oil is also rich in antioxidants, which can help to protect the skin from damage.

Jojoba Oil - Jojoba oil is another popular lubricant used in Gua Sha practice. It is similar in texture to the natural oils produced by the skin, which can make it more easily absorbed and less likely to clog pores. Jojoba oil is also rich in vitamins and minerals, which can help to nourish and protect the skin.

Grapeseed Oil - Grapeseed oil is a light, non-greasy oil that is commonly used in Gua Sha practice. It is easily absorbed by the skin and can help to reduce inflammation and redness. Grapeseed oil is also rich in antioxidants, which can help to protect the skin from damage.

Sweet Almond Oil - Sweet almond oil is a gentle, nourishing oil that is commonly used in Gua Sha practice. It is rich in vitamins and minerals, which can help to soothe and hydrate the skin. Sweet almond oil is also non-comedogenic, which means it is less likely to clog pores.

Sunflower Oil - Sunflower oil is a light, non-greasy oil that is commonly used in Gua Sha practice. It is easily absorbed by the skin and can help to moisturize and protect the skin. Sunflower oil is also rich in vitamin E, which can help to reduce inflammation and promote healthy skin.

Choosing the Right Lubricant or Oil

When choosing a lubricant or oil for Gua Sha practice, it is important to consider the specific needs of the individual and the condition being treated. For example, someone with dry or sensitive skin may benefit from a heavier, more moisturizing oil, while someone with oily or acne-prone skin may benefit from a lighter, non-greasy oil.

It is also important to choose high-quality oils and lubricants that are free from synthetic fragrances, preservatives, and other harmful ingredients. Look for products that are labeled as organic, natural, or pure, and avoid products that contain synthetic chemicals or additives.

Using Lubricants and Oils in Gua Sha Practice

When using lubricants and oils in Gua Sha practice, it is important to use them sparingly and to avoid applying too much pressure. Too much lubricant can cause the tool to slip and slide on the skin, which can reduce the effectiveness of the treatment. It can also make it difficult to apply the right amount of pressure, which can increase the risk of bruising or damage.

To use a lubricant or oil in Gua Sha practice, simply apply a small amount to the area being treated and massage it into the skin. Use the tool to scrape the skin in a firm and repetitive manner, being careful not to apply too much pressure or cause too much friction.

Chapter Three

# Preparing for a Gua Sha Session

Gua Sha is a traditional Chinese medicine technique that involves using a smooth-edged tool to scrape the skin in a firm and repetitive manner. Proper preparation is important before a Gua Sha session to ensure that the treatment is safe and effective. Below we will explore some tips for preparing for a Gua Sha session.

Hydrate and Nourish the Skin

Before a Gua Sha session, it is important to hydrate and nourish the skin. This can help to make the skin more pliable and receptive to the treatment. Some ways to hydrate and nourish the skin before a Gua Sha session include:

Drinking plenty of water - Drinking water can help to hydrate the skin from the inside out, making it more supple and resilient.

Applying a moisturizer - Applying a moisturizer can help to nourish the skin and make it more receptive to the Gua Sha tool. Look for a moisturizer that is free from synthetic fragrances, preservatives, and other harmful ingredients.

Using a facial oil - Using a facial oil can help to nourish and protect the skin, making it more receptive to the Gua Sha tool. Look for an oil that is light and non-greasy, and free from synthetic chemicals and additives.

Prepare the Gua Sha Tool and Materials

Before a Gua Sha session, it is important to prepare the Gua Sha tool and materials. This can help to ensure that the treatment is safe and effective. Some ways to prepare the Gua Sha tool and materials include:

Disinfecting the Gua Sha tool - Disinfect the Gua Sha tool before and after use to prevent the spread of bacteria and other pathogens. Use a cleaning solution, such as rubbing alcohol, to disinfect the tool.

Preparing the lubricant - Prepare the lubricant before the Gua Sha session to ensure that it is ready when needed. Choose a high-quality lubricant, such as coconut oil or jojoba oil, that is free from synthetic fragrances and additives.

Gathering towels and other materials - Gather towels and other materials, such as disposable gloves, that may be needed during the Gua Sha session. Make sure that everything is clean and ready to use.

Prepare Yourself Mentally and Emotionally

Before a Gua Sha session, it is important to prepare yourself mentally and emotionally. This can help to ensure that you are relaxed and open to the treatment. Some ways to prepare yourself mentally and emotionally include:

Setting an intention - Set an intention for the Gua Sha session, such as relaxation, healing, or rejuvenation. This can help to focus your mind and create a positive mindset.

Breathing deeply - Take a few deep breaths before the Gua Sha session to help relax your body and mind.

Visualizing the outcome - Visualize the outcome of the Gua Sha session, such as reduced pain, improved circulation, or a brighter complexion.

This can help to create a positive mindset and make the treatment more effective.

## Creating a comfortable environment

Gua Sha is a traditional Chinese medicine technique that involves using a smooth-edged tool to scrape the skin in a firm and repetitive manner. Creating a comfortable environment is an important aspect of Gua Sha practice, as it can help to enhance the benefits of the treatment and leave the individual feeling relaxed and rejuvenated. Below we will explore some tips for creating a comfortable environment for Gua Sha practice.

Choosing a Comfortable Space

When preparing for a Gua Sha session, it is important to choose a comfortable space that is free from distractions and interruptions. The space should be quiet and peaceful, with minimal noise and distractions. It should also be well-ventilated, with good air circulation and temperature control.

Some tips for choosing a comfortable space for Gua Sha practice include:

Choosing a quiet space - Choose a space that is free from noise and distractions, such as a quiet room in your home or a private treatment room at a spa or wellness center.

Controlling the temperature - Make sure that the space is at a comfortable temperature, neither too hot nor too cold. This can help to enhance the benefits of the treatment and leave the individual feeling relaxed and comfortable.

Ensuring good air circulation - Make sure that the space is well-ventilated, with good air circulation. This can help to prevent the buildup of stale air and ensure that the individual is breathing fresh, clean air during the treatment.

Creating a Relaxing Atmosphere

Creating a relaxing atmosphere is another important aspect of Gua Sha practice. This can help to enhance the benefits of the treatment and leave the individual feeling calm and relaxed. Some tips for creating a relaxing atmosphere for Gua Sha practice include:

Using soothing lighting - Use soft, dim lighting to create a relaxing atmosphere. Avoid bright, harsh lights that can be jarring and disruptive.

Playing calming music - Play soft, calming music to help the individual relax and unwind. Avoid music with a strong beat or loud, jarring sounds.

Using aromatherapy - Use essential oils or aromatherapy diffusers to create a relaxing atmosphere. Lavender, chamomile, and ylang-ylang are all popular essential oils for relaxation.

Providing Comfortable Equipment and Materials

Providing comfortable equipment and materials is another important aspect of Gua Sha practice. This can help to enhance the benefits of the treatment and leave the individual feeling comfortable and relaxed. Some tips for providing comfortable equipment and materials for Gua Sha practice include:

Using a comfortable massage table - Use a comfortable massage table or treatment bed that is padded and supportive. This can help to reduce pressure points and ensure that the individual is comfortable throughout the treatment.

Providing comfortable pillows and bolsters - Provide comfortable pillows and bolsters to help support the individual's head, neck, and back during the treatment. This can help to reduce tension and discomfort.

Using soft, comfortable linens - Use soft, comfortable linens, such as clean sheets and blankets, to cover the massage table or treatment bed. This can help to create a comfortable and relaxing atmosphere.

## Contraindications and safety precautions

Gua Sha is a traditional Chinese medicine technique that involves using a smooth-edged tool to scrape the skin in a firm and repetitive manner. While Gua Sha is generally safe and effective when performed correctly, there are some contraindications and safety precautions that should be taken into account to ensure that the treatment is safe for the individual. Below we will explore some of the contraindications and safety precautions for Gua Sha practice.

Contraindications for Gua Sha

Contraindications are medical conditions or situations in which Gua Sha should not be performed. Some contraindications for Gua Sha include:

Skin conditions - Gua Sha should not be performed on areas of the skin that are irritated, inflamed, or infected. This can include conditions such as eczema, psoriasis, and acne.

Broken skin - Gua Sha should not be performed on areas of the skin that are broken or have open wounds, as this can increase the risk of infection.

Recent surgeries - Gua Sha should not be performed on areas of the body that have recently undergone surgery or have stitches, as this can disrupt the healing process.

Blood disorders - Gua Sha should not be performed on individuals with blood disorders, such as hemophilia, as this can increase the risk of bleeding and bruising.

Pregnancy - Gua Sha should not be performed on pregnant women, particularly on the abdomen, as this can stimulate contractions and increase the risk of miscarriage.

Safety Precautions for Gua Sha

In addition to contraindications, there are also some safety precautions that should be taken into account when performing Gua Sha. Some safety precautions for Gua Sha include:

Using a clean and sterilized tool - The Gua Sha tool should be clean and sterilized before each use to prevent the spread of bacteria and other pathogens.

Using a lubricant - A lubricant, such as coconut oil or jojoba oil, should be used to help the tool glide smoothly over the skin and prevent bruising or damage.

Avoiding excessive pressure - Excessive pressure should be avoided during Gua Sha, as this can increase the risk of bruising, damage, and pain.

Checking for signs of discomfort - The individual should be checked for signs of discomfort during Gua Sha, such as pain, redness, or swelling. If these signs are present, the treatment should be stopped immediately.

Following up after treatment - The individual should be checked and followed up with after the Gua Sha treatment to ensure that they are not experiencing any adverse reactions or complications.

Chapter Four

# Gua Sha Techniques and Strokes

Gua Sha is a traditional Chinese medicine technique that involves using a smooth-edged tool to scrape the skin in a firm and repetitive manner. The technique is used to promote healing, reduce pain, improve circulation, and enhance overall well-being. Below we will explore some of the Gua Sha techniques and strokes that are used in practice.

Basic Gua Sha Techniques

The basic Gua Sha technique involves using a smooth-edged tool to apply pressure to the skin and scrape it in a firm and repetitive manner. The tool is held at a 45-degree angle to the skin, and pressure is applied in the direction of the lymphatic flow. Some basic Gua Sha techniques include:

Short strokes - Short strokes are used to scrape the skin in a rapid and repetitive manner, typically in an up-and-down or back-and-forth motion. This technique is often used to promote circulation and reduce pain.

Long strokes - Long strokes are used to scrape the skin in a slower and more deliberate manner, typically in a single direction. This technique is often used to promote lymphatic drainage and detoxification.

Circular strokes - Circular strokes are used to scrape the skin in a circular motion, typically in a small area. This technique is often used to promote healing and reduce inflammation.

Advanced Gua Sha Techniques

In addition to the basic techniques, there are also some more advanced Gua Sha techniques that are used in practice. These techniques may require additional training and experience, and should only be performed by a trained and qualified practitioner. Some advanced Gua Sha techniques include:

Three-dimensional strokes - Three-dimensional strokes involve scraping the skin in multiple directions and angles, creating a three-dimensional effect. This technique is often used to promote deep tissue healing and rejuvenation.

Meridian strokes - Meridian strokes involve following the meridian lines of the body, which are the energy channels that run throughout the body. This technique is often used to balance the body's energy and promote overall wellness.

Facial Gua Sha - Facial Gua Sha is a specialized technique that involves using a smooth-edged tool to massage and scrape the skin on the face and neck. This technique is often used to promote circulation, reduce wrinkles and fine lines, and improve the overall appearance of the skin.

Safety Considerations

While Gua Sha is generally safe and effective when performed correctly, there are some safety considerations that should be taken into account to ensure that the treatment is safe for the individual. Some safety considerations for Gua Sha include:

Avoiding bony areas - Gua Sha should not be performed on bony areas, such as the spine or the shoulder blades, as this can increase the risk of bruising, damage, and pain.

Avoiding sensitive areas - Gua Sha should not be performed on sensitive areas, such as the face, genitals, or breasts, as this can cause discomfort or pain.

Following up after treatment - The individual should be checked and followed up with after the Gua Sha treatment to ensure that they are not experiencing any adverse reactions or complications.

## Basic strokes

Gua Sha is a traditional Chinese medicine technique that involves using a smooth-edged tool to scrape the skin in a firm and repetitive manner. The technique is used to promote healing, reduce pain, improve circulation, and enhance overall well-being. Below we will explore some of the basic Gua Sha strokes that are used in practice.

Short Strokes

Short strokes are one of the most basic Gua Sha techniques. This technique involves using a smooth-edged tool to scrape the skin in a rapid and repetitive manner, typically in an up-and-down or back-and-forth motion. Short strokes are often used to promote circulation and reduce pain.

To perform short strokes, the practitioner holds the tool at a 45-degree angle to the skin, and applies pressure in the direction of the lymphatic flow. The strokes should be short, rapid, and repetitive, and should cover a small area of the skin at a time. The pressure should be firm but not too intense, and should be adjusted based on the individual's tolerance and sensitivity.

Long Strokes

Long strokes are another basic Gua Sha technique. This technique involves using a smooth-edged tool to scrape the skin in a slower and more deliberate manner, typically in a single direction. Long strokes are often used to promote lymphatic drainage and detoxification.

To perform long strokes, the practitioner holds the tool at a 45-degree angle to the skin, and applies pressure in the direction of the lymphatic flow. The strokes should be slow and deliberate, and should cover a larger area of the skin at a time. The pressure should be firm but not too intense, and should be adjusted based on the individual's tolerance and sensitivity.

Circular Strokes

Circular strokes are another basic Gua Sha technique. This technique involves using a smooth-edged tool to scrape the skin in a circular motion, typically in a small area. Circular strokes are often used to promote healing and reduce inflammation.

To perform circular strokes, the practitioner holds the tool at a 45-degree angle to the skin, and applies pressure in a circular motion. The strokes should be slow and deliberate, and should cover a small area of the skin at a time. The pressure should be firm but not too intense, and should be adjusted based on the individual's tolerance and sensitivity.

Combination Strokes

Combination strokes are a more advanced Gua Sha technique that involves combining different strokes to create a more complex treatment. Combination strokes can be used to target specific areas of the body or to address specific health concerns.

To perform combination strokes, the practitioner combines different stroke techniques, such as short strokes, long strokes, and circular strokes, to create a customized treatment. The strokes should be adjusted based on the individual's tolerance and sensitivity, and should be tailored to address their specific health concerns.

## Advanced techniques

Gua Sha is a traditional Chinese medicine technique that involves using a smooth-edged tool to scrape the skin in a firm and repetitive manner. The technique is used to promote healing, reduce pain, improve circulation, and enhance overall well-being. In addition to basic strokes, there are also some advanced Gua Sha techniques that are used in practice. Below we will explore some of the advanced Gua Sha techniques.

Three-Dimensional Strokes

Three-dimensional strokes are an advanced Gua Sha technique that involves scraping the skin in multiple directions and angles, creating a three-dimensional effect. This technique is often used to promote deep tissue healing and rejuvenation.

To perform three-dimensional strokes, the practitioner holds the tool at a 45-degree angle to the skin, and applies pressure in multiple directions and angles. The strokes should be slow and deliberate, and should cover a larger area of the skin at a time. The pressure should be firm but not too intense, and should be adjusted based on the individual's tolerance and sensitivity.

Meridian Strokes

Meridian strokes are another advanced Gua Sha technique that involves following the meridian lines of the body, which are the energy channels that run throughout the body. This technique is often used to balance the body's energy and promote overall wellness.

To perform meridian strokes, the practitioner follows the meridian lines of the body, using the Gua Sha tool to apply pressure and scrape the skin along the energy channels. The strokes should be slow and deliberate, and should be adjusted based on the individual's tolerance and sensitivity.

Facial Gua Sha

Facial Gua Sha is a specialized Gua Sha technique that involves using a smooth-edged tool to massage and scrape the skin on the face and neck. This technique is often used to promote circulation, reduce wrinkles and fine lines, and improve the overall appearance of the skin.

To perform facial Gua Sha, the practitioner uses a smaller and more delicate Gua Sha tool, and applies pressure and scraping motions to the skin on the face and neck. The strokes should be gentle and controlled, and should be adjusted based on the individual's tolerance and sensitivity.

Chapter Five

# Gua Sha for the Face

Gua Sha is a traditional Chinese medicine technique that involves using a smooth-edged tool to scrape the skin in a firm and repetitive manner. While Gua Sha is often used on the body for pain relief and circulation, it is also gaining popularity as a facial treatment. Below we will explore the benefits and techniques of using Gua Sha for the face.

Benefits of Gua Sha for the Face

Gua Sha for the face offers a range of benefits for the skin and overall well-being. Some of the benefits include:

Improving circulation - Gua Sha for the face can improve circulation to the skin, which can help to promote a healthy glow and reduce puffiness and dark circles.

Reducing wrinkles and fine lines - Gua Sha for the face can help to reduce wrinkles and fine lines by promoting collagen production and improving circulation.

Relieving tension - Gua Sha for the face can help to relieve tension in the facial muscles, which can reduce stress and promote relaxation.

Promoting lymphatic drainage - Gua Sha for the face can promote lymphatic drainage, which can help to reduce puffiness and promote a more even skin tone.

Enhancing product absorption - Gua Sha for the face can enhance the absorption of skincare products, allowing them to penetrate deeper into the skin for more effective results.

Gua Sha Techniques for the Face

Gua Sha for the face involves using a smaller and more delicate tool than the ones used on the body. The tool is typically made from rose quartz, jade, or other smooth and cool stones, which can provide additional benefits for the skin.

To perform Gua Sha for the face, the practitioner uses the tool to apply pressure and scraping motions to the skin on the face and neck. The strokes should be gentle and controlled, and should be adjusted based on the individual's tolerance and sensitivity. Some basic Gua Sha techniques for the face include:

Forehead - Starting at the center of the forehead, use the tool to scrape outward and upward towards the hairline.

Cheeks - Starting at the nose, use the tool to scrape outward and upward towards the ears.

Jawline - Starting at the chin, use the tool to scrape outward and upward towards the ears.

Neck - Starting at the base of the neck, use the tool to scrape upward towards the chin.

It is important to note that Gua Sha for the face should be performed by a trained and qualified practitioner, or under their guidance. The technique should be performed gently and without causing pain or discomfort to the individual.

## Facial rejuvenation

Facial rejuvenation is a popular area of interest for many people, especially as they age and begin to notice changes in their skin. While there are many treatments available, including invasive procedures such as surgery or injections, there are also more natural and holistic options, such as Gua Sha. Below we will explore how Gua Sha can be used for facial rejuvenation.

What is Facial Rejuvenation?

Facial rejuvenation is the process of restoring the skin's youthful appearance and vitality. This can include reducing the appearance of fine lines and wrinkles, improving skin texture and tone, and promoting a healthy glow. Facial rejuvenation can be achieved through a variety of treatments, including skincare products, facial exercises, and non-invasive procedures such as Gua Sha.

How Does Gua Sha Work for Facial Rejuvenation?

Gua Sha is a traditional Chinese medicine technique that involves using a smooth-edged tool to scrape the skin in a firm and repetitive manner. When used for facial rejuvenation, Gua Sha can promote lymphatic drainage, increase circulation, and reduce tension in the facial muscles. These benefits can help to reduce puffiness, fine lines, and wrinkles, and promote a more youthful and vibrant appearance.

Gua Sha for facial rejuvenation involves using a smaller and more delicate tool than the ones used on the body. The tool is typically made from rose quartz, jade, or other smooth and cool stones, which can provide additional benefits for the skin. The practitioner uses the tool to apply pressure and scraping motions to the skin on the face and neck, using a variety of techniques and strokes to promote lymphatic drainage, increase circulation, and reduce tension.

Benefits of Gua Sha for Facial Rejuvenation

There are many benefits to using Gua Sha for facial rejuvenation, including:

Promoting lymphatic drainage - Gua Sha can promote lymphatic drainage in the face, reducing puffiness and promoting a more even skin tone.

Increasing circulation - Gua Sha can increase circulation to the face, promoting a healthy glow and improving the skin's overall appearance.

Reducing tension - Gua Sha can reduce tension in the facial muscles, promoting relaxation and reducing the appearance of fine lines and wrinkles.

Improving product absorption - Gua Sha can improve the absorption of skincare products, allowing them to penetrate deeper into the skin for more effective results.

Promoting overall wellness - Gua Sha is a holistic technique that can promote overall well-being, reducing stress and promoting relaxation.

Gua Sha Techniques for Facial Rejuvenation

Some of the Gua Sha techniques used for facial rejuvenation include:

Forehead - Starting at the center of the forehead, use the tool to scrape outward and upward towards the hairline.

Cheeks - Starting at the nose, use the tool to scrape outward and upward towards the ears.

Jawline - Starting at the chin, use the tool to scrape outward and upward towards the ears.

Neck - Starting at the base of the neck, use the tool to scrape upward towards the chin.

It is important to note that Gua Sha for facial rejuvenation should be performed by a trained and qualified practitioner, or under their guidance. The technique should be performed gently and without causing pain or discomfort to the individual.

## Sinus relief and headache reduction

Sinus congestion and headaches are common ailments that can be caused by a variety of factors, such as allergies, colds, and stress. While there are many treatments available, including medications and nasal sprays, there are also natural and holistic options, such as Gua Sha. Below we will explore how Gua Sha can be used for sinus relief and headache reduction.

What is Gua Sha?

Gua Sha is a traditional Chinese medicine technique that involves using a smooth-edged tool to scrape the skin in a firm and repetitive manner. The technique is used to promote healing, reduce pain, improve circulation, and enhance overall well-being. Gua Sha is typically used on the body, but can also be used on the face and head for specific conditions.

How Does Gua Sha Work for Sinus Relief and Headache Reduction?

Gua Sha for sinus relief and headache reduction involves using the Gua Sha tool to apply pressure and scraping motions to specific points on the head and face. These points are located along the meridian lines of the body, which are the energy channels that run throughout the body. By stimulating these points, Gua Sha can promote the flow of energy and relieve congestion, reducing sinus pressure and headaches.

Benefits of Gua Sha for Sinus Relief and Headache Reduction

There are many benefits to using Gua Sha for sinus relief and headache reduction, including:

Reducing sinus congestion - Gua Sha can promote the flow of energy and relieve congestion in the sinuses, reducing sinus pressure and congestion.

Relieving headaches - Gua Sha can help to relieve tension in the muscles and promote relaxation, reducing the frequency and intensity of headaches.

Promoting relaxation - Gua Sha is a holistic technique that can promote overall well-being and relaxation, reducing stress and tension in the body.

Reducing inflammation - Gua Sha can help to reduce inflammation in the body, which can contribute to sinus congestion and headaches.

Gua Sha Techniques for Sinus Relief and Headache Reduction

Some of the Gua Sha techniques used for sinus relief and headache reduction include:

Temple - Starting at the temples, use the Gua Sha tool to scrape downward towards the cheekbones.

Sinuses - Starting at the bridge of the nose, use the Gua Sha tool to scrape outward and upward towards the temples.

Neck - Starting at the base of the neck, use the Gua Sha tool to scrape upward towards the base of the skull.

Scalp - Use the Gua Sha tool to gently scrape the scalp in a circular motion, focusing on areas where tension and headaches are present.

It is important to note that Gua Sha for sinus relief and headache reduction should be performed by a trained and qualified practitioner, or under their guidance. The technique should be performed gently and without causing pain or discomfort to the individual.

Chapter Six

# Gua Sha for the Neck and Shoulders

Gua Sha is a traditional Chinese medicine technique that involves using a smooth-edged tool to scrape the skin in a firm and repetitive manner. The technique is commonly used for pain relief, circulation improvement, and relaxation. Below we will explore how Gua Sha can be used for the neck and shoulders.

Neck and Shoulder Pain

Neck and shoulder pain is a common complaint, especially among people who sit at desks or engage in repetitive motions for extended periods of time. This type of pain can be caused by a variety of factors, including poor posture, stress, and injury. While there are many treatments available, including medications, physical therapy, and massage, there are also natural and holistic options, such as Gua Sha.

How Does Gua Sha Work for the Neck and Shoulders?

Gua Sha for the neck and shoulders involves using the Gua Sha tool to apply pressure and scraping motions to specific points on the neck and shoulders. These points are located along the meridian lines of the body, which are the energy channels that run throughout the body. By stimulating these points, Gua Sha can promote the flow of energy and reduce pain and tension in the neck and shoulders.

Benefits of Gua Sha for the Neck and Shoulders

There are many benefits to using Gua Sha for the neck and shoulders, including:

Reducing pain and tension - Gua Sha can help to reduce pain and tension in the neck and shoulders, promoting relaxation and reducing discomfort.

Improving circulation - Gua Sha can improve circulation in the neck and shoulders, promoting healing and reducing inflammation.

Reducing inflammation - Gua Sha can help to reduce inflammation in the neck and shoulders, which can contribute to pain and discomfort.

Promoting relaxation - Gua Sha is a holistic technique that can promote overall well-being and relaxation, reducing stress and tension in the body.

Gua Sha Techniques for the Neck and Shoulders

Some of the Gua Sha techniques used for the neck and shoulders include:

Base of the Neck - Starting at the base of the neck, use the Gua Sha tool to scrape upward towards the base of the skull.

Shoulders - Starting at the top of the shoulders, use the Gua Sha tool to scrape outward towards the edges of the shoulders.

Upper Back - Use the Gua Sha tool to scrape the upper back in a downward motion towards the waist.

Trapezius Muscle - Use the Gua Sha tool to scrape the trapezius muscle, which is located at the top of the shoulders, in an upward and outward motion towards the shoulders.

It is important to note that Gua Sha for the neck and shoulders should be performed by a trained and qualified practitioner, or under their guidance.

The technique should be performed gently and without causing pain or discomfort to the individual.

## Tension relief

Tension is a common problem for many people, whether it is caused by stress, poor posture, or physical exertion. While there are many treatments available, including massage, physical therapy, and medication, there are also natural and holistic options, such as Gua Sha. Below we will explore how Gua Sha can be used for tension relief.

What is Tension?

Tension is a feeling of tightness or strain in the muscles, often caused by stress, anxiety, or physical exertion. Tension can be experienced in any part of the body, but is most commonly felt in the neck, shoulders, and back.

How Does Gua Sha Work for Tension Relief?

Gua Sha for tension relief involves using the Gua Sha tool to apply pressure and scraping motions to specific points on the body. These points are located along the meridian lines of the body, which are the energy channels that run throughout the body. By stimulating these points, Gua Sha can promote the flow of energy and reduce tension and tightness in the muscles.

Benefits of Gua Sha for Tension Relief

There are many benefits to using Gua Sha for tension relief, including:

Reducing muscle tension - Gua Sha can help to reduce tension in the muscles, promoting relaxation and reducing discomfort.

Improving circulation - Gua Sha can improve circulation in the body, promoting healing and reducing inflammation.

Promoting relaxation - Gua Sha is a holistic technique that can promote overall well-being and relaxation, reducing stress and tension in the body.

Reducing inflammation - Gua Sha can help to reduce inflammation in the body, which can contribute to tension and discomfort.

Gua Sha Techniques for Tension Relief

Some of the Gua Sha techniques used for tension relief include:

Neck - Starting at the base of the neck, use the Gua Sha tool to scrape upward towards the base of the skull.

Shoulders - Starting at the top of the shoulders, use the Gua Sha tool to scrape outward towards the edges of the shoulders.

Back - Use the Gua Sha tool to scrape the back in a downward motion towards the waist.

Legs - Use the Gua Sha tool to scrape the legs in an upward motion towards the hips.

It is important to note that Gua Sha for tension relief should be performed by a trained and qualified practitioner, or under their guidance. The technique should be performed gently and without causing pain or discomfort to the individual.

## Posture improvement

Posture is an essential aspect of good health and well-being. Poor posture can lead to a variety of problems, including back pain, neck pain, headaches, and fatigue. While there are many treatments available, including physical therapy and chiropractic adjustments, there are also natural and holistic options, such as Gua Sha. Below we will explore how Gua Sha can be used to improve posture.

What is Posture?

Posture is the way in which we hold our bodies, including the position of the spine, shoulders, and hips. Good posture involves aligning these body parts in a way that allows for optimal function and movement.

How Does Gua Sha Work for Posture Improvement?

Gua Sha for posture improvement involves using the Gua Sha tool to apply pressure and scraping motions to specific points on the body. These points are located along the meridian lines of the body, which are the energy channels that run throughout the body. By stimulating these points, Gua Sha can promote the flow of energy and help to align the body in a way that promotes good posture.

Benefits of Gua Sha for Posture Improvement

There are many benefits to using Gua Sha for posture improvement, including:

Reducing muscle tension - Gua Sha can help to reduce tension in the muscles, promoting relaxation and reducing discomfort.

Improving alignment - Gua Sha can help to align the body in a way that promotes good posture and optimal function.

Promoting relaxation - Gua Sha is a holistic technique that can promote overall well-being and relaxation, reducing stress and tension in the body.

Reducing inflammation - Gua Sha can help to reduce inflammation in the body, which can contribute to poor posture and discomfort.

Gua Sha Techniques for Posture Improvement

Some of the Gua Sha techniques used for posture improvement include:

Upper Back - Use the Gua Sha tool to scrape the upper back in a downward motion towards the waist.

Shoulders - Starting at the top of the shoulders, use the Gua Sha tool to scrape outward towards the edges of the shoulders.

Neck - Starting at the base of the neck, use the Gua Sha tool to scrape upward towards the base of the skull.

Hips - Use the Gua Sha tool to scrape the hips in a circular motion, focusing on areas where tension and discomfort are present.

It is important to note that Gua Sha for posture improvement should be performed by a trained and qualified practitioner, or under their guidance. The technique should be performed gently and without causing pain or discomfort to the individual.

Chapter Seven

# Gua Sha for the Upper Back

Gua Sha is a traditional Chinese medicine technique that has been used for centuries to relieve pain, improve circulation, and promote relaxation. The technique involves using a smooth-edged tool to scrape the skin in a firm and repetitive manner. Below we will explore how Gua Sha can be used for the upper back.

Upper Back Pain

Upper back pain is a common problem for many people, whether it is caused by poor posture, stress, or injury. This type of pain can be debilitating and can interfere with daily activities. While there are many treatments available, including medications, physical therapy, and massage, there are also natural and holistic options, such as Gua Sha.

How Does Gua Sha Work for the Upper Back?

Gua Sha for the upper back involves using the Gua Sha tool to apply pressure and scraping motions to specific points on the upper back. These points are located along the meridian lines of the body, which are the energy channels that run throughout the body. By stimulating these points, Gua Sha can promote the flow of energy and reduce pain and tension in the upper back.

Benefits of Gua Sha for the Upper Back

There are many benefits to using Gua Sha for the upper back, including:

Reducing pain and tension - Gua Sha can help to reduce pain and tension in the upper back, promoting relaxation and reducing discomfort.

Improving circulation - Gua Sha can improve circulation in the upper back, promoting healing and reducing inflammation.

Reducing inflammation - Gua Sha can help to reduce inflammation in the upper back, which can contribute to pain and discomfort.

Promoting relaxation - Gua Sha is a holistic technique that can promote overall well-being and relaxation, reducing stress and tension in the body.

Gua Sha Techniques for the Upper Back

Some of the Gua Sha techniques used for the upper back include:

The Trapezius Muscle - Use the Gua Sha tool to scrape the trapezius muscle, which is located at the top of the shoulders, in an upward and outward motion towards the shoulders.

The Rhomboid Muscles - Use the Gua Sha tool to scrape the rhomboid muscles, which are located between the shoulder blades, in a downward motion towards the waist.

The Scapula - Use the Gua Sha tool to scrape the scapula, which is the bone that connects the shoulder blade to the collarbone, in a circular motion.

The Upper Spine - Use the Gua Sha tool to scrape the upper spine in a downward motion towards the waist.

It is important to note that Gua Sha for the upper back should be performed by a trained and qualified practitioner, or under their guidance. The technique should be performed gently and without causing pain or discomfort to the individual.

## Relieving back pain

Back pain is a common problem for many people, and it can be caused by a variety of factors, including poor posture, injury, and stress. While there are many treatments available, including medications, physical therapy, and chiropractic adjustments, there are also natural and holistic options, such as Gua Sha. Below we will explore how Gua Sha can be used to relieve back pain.

What is Back Pain?

Back pain is a common problem that can affect people of all ages. It can be caused by a variety of factors, including poor posture, injury, and stress. Back pain can be acute, which means it is sudden and severe, or chronic, which means it lasts for a longer period of time.

How Does Gua Sha Work for Back Pain Relief?

Gua Sha for back pain relief involves using the Gua Sha tool to apply pressure and scraping motions to specific points on the back. These points are located along the meridian lines of the body, which are the energy channels that run throughout the body. By stimulating these points, Gua Sha can promote the flow of energy and reduce pain and tension in the back.

Benefits of Gua Sha for Back Pain Relief

There are many benefits to using Gua Sha for back pain relief, including:

Reducing pain and tension - Gua Sha can help to reduce pain and tension in the back, promoting relaxation and reducing discomfort.

Improving circulation - Gua Sha can improve circulation in the back, promoting healing and reducing inflammation.

Reducing inflammation - Gua Sha can help to reduce inflammation in the back, which can contribute to pain and discomfort.

Promoting relaxation - Gua Sha is a holistic technique that can promote overall well-being and relaxation, reducing stress and tension in the body.

Gua Sha Techniques for Back Pain Relief

Some of the Gua Sha techniques used for back pain relief include:

Lower Back - Use the Gua Sha tool to scrape the lower back in an upward motion towards the waist.

Upper Back - Use the Gua Sha tool to scrape the upper back in a downward motion towards the waist.

Shoulders - Use the Gua Sha tool to scrape the shoulders in an outward motion towards the arms.

Hips - Use the Gua Sha tool to scrape the hips in a circular motion, focusing on areas where tension and discomfort are present.

It is important to note that Gua Sha for back pain relief should be performed by a trained and qualified practitioner, or under their guidance. The technique should be performed gently and without causing pain or discomfort to the individual.

## Enhancing respiratory health

Respiratory health is essential for overall well-being, and it can be affected by a variety of factors, including environmental pollutants, allergies, and infections. While there are many treatments available, including medications, inhalers, and breathing exercises, there are also natural and holistic options, such as Gua Sha. Below we will explore how Gua Sha can be used to enhance respiratory health.

What is Gua Sha?

Gua Sha is a traditional Chinese medicine technique that involves using a smooth-edged tool to scrape the skin in a firm and repetitive manner. The technique is used to stimulate the flow of energy, or Qi, throughout the body, and it is often used to promote relaxation, relieve pain, and improve circulation.

How Does Gua Sha Work for Enhancing Respiratory Health?

Gua Sha for enhancing respiratory health involves using the Gua Sha tool to apply pressure and scraping motions to specific points on the back, chest, and neck. These points are located along the meridian lines of the body, which are the energy channels that run throughout the body. By stimulating these points, Gua Sha can promote the flow of energy and reduce tension in the respiratory muscles, allowing for deeper and more efficient breathing.

Benefits of Gua Sha for Enhancing Respiratory Health

There are many benefits to using Gua Sha for enhancing respiratory health, including:

Reducing tension in the respiratory muscles - Gua Sha can help to reduce tension in the muscles used for breathing, promoting more efficient and deeper breathing.

Improving lung function - Gua Sha can improve lung function by promoting better airflow and oxygenation.

Reducing inflammation - Gua Sha can help to reduce inflammation in the respiratory system, which can contribute to respiratory problems.

Promoting relaxation - Gua Sha is a holistic technique that can promote overall well-being and relaxation, reducing stress and tension in the body.

Gua Sha Techniques for Enhancing Respiratory Health

Some of the Gua Sha techniques used for enhancing respiratory health include:

Back - Use the Gua Sha tool to scrape the back in an upward motion towards the shoulders, focusing on areas where tension and discomfort are present.

Chest - Use the Gua Sha tool to scrape the chest in a downward motion towards the waist, focusing on the areas around the lungs.

Neck - Use the Gua Sha tool to scrape the sides of the neck in a downward motion towards the shoulders, focusing on the areas around the lymph nodes.

Upper Back - Use the Gua Sha tool to scrape the upper back in a circular motion, focusing on areas where tension and discomfort are present.

It is important to note that Gua Sha for enhancing respiratory health should be performed by a trained and qualified practitioner, or under their guidance. The technique should be performed gently and without causing pain or discomfort to the individual.

Chapter Eight

# Gua Sha for the Lower Back and Hips

The lower back and hips are areas of the body that can be particularly susceptible to tension and pain. This can be caused by a variety of factors, including poor posture, injury, and stress. While there are many treatments available, including medications, physical therapy, and chiropractic adjustments, there are also natural and holistic options, such as Gua Sha. Below we will explore how Gua Sha can be used to alleviate pain and tension in the lower back and hips.

What is Gua Sha?

Gua Sha is a traditional Chinese medicine technique that involves using a smooth-edged tool to scrape the skin in a firm and repetitive manner. The technique is used to stimulate the flow of energy, or Qi, throughout the body, and it is often used to promote relaxation, relieve pain, and improve circulation.

How Does Gua Sha Work for the Lower Back and Hips?

Gua Sha for the lower back and hips involves using the Gua Sha tool to apply pressure and scraping motions to specific points on the back, hips, and glutes. These points are located along the meridian lines of the body, which are the energy channels that run throughout the body. By stimulating these points, Gua Sha can promote the flow of energy and reduce pain and tension in the lower back and hips.

Benefits of Gua Sha for the Lower Back and Hips

There are many benefits to using Gua Sha for the lower back and hips, including:

Reducing pain and tension - Gua Sha can help to reduce pain and tension in the lower back and hips, promoting relaxation and reducing discomfort.

Improving circulation - Gua Sha can improve circulation in the lower back and hips, promoting healing and reducing inflammation.

Reducing inflammation - Gua Sha can help to reduce inflammation in the lower back and hips, which can contribute to pain and discomfort.

Promoting relaxation - Gua Sha is a holistic technique that can promote overall well-being and relaxation, reducing stress and tension in the body.

Gua Sha Techniques for the Lower Back and Hips

Some of the Gua Sha techniques used for the lower back and hips include:

Lower Back - Use the Gua Sha tool to scrape the lower back in an upward motion towards the waist, focusing on areas where tension and discomfort are present.

Hips - Use the Gua Sha tool to scrape the hips in a circular motion, focusing on areas where tension and discomfort are present.

Glutes - Use the Gua Sha tool to scrape the glutes in an upward motion towards the waist, focusing on areas where tension and discomfort are present.

IT Band - Use the Gua Sha tool to scrape the IT band in a downward motion towards the knee, focusing on areas where tension and discomfort are present.

It is important to note that Gua Sha for the lower back and hips should be performed by a trained and qualified practitioner, or under their guidance. The technique should be performed gently and without causing pain or discomfort to the individual.

## Addressing lower back pain

Lower back pain is a common condition that affects many people worldwide. It can be caused by a variety of factors, including poor posture, injury, and stress. While there are many treatments available, including medications, physical therapy, and chiropractic adjustments, there are also natural and holistic options, such as Gua Sha. Below we will explore how Gua Sha can be used to address lower back pain.

What is Gua Sha?

Gua Sha is a traditional Chinese medicine technique that involves using a smooth-edged tool to scrape the skin in a firm and repetitive manner. The technique is used to stimulate the flow of energy, or Qi, throughout the body, and it is often used to promote relaxation, relieve pain, and improve circulation.

How Does Gua Sha Work for Lower Back Pain?

Gua Sha for lower back pain involves using the Gua Sha tool to apply pressure and scraping motions to specific points on the lower back. These points are located along the meridian lines of the body, which are the energy channels that run throughout the body. By stimulating these points, Gua Sha can promote the flow of energy and reduce pain and tension in the lower back.

Benefits of Gua Sha for Lower Back Pain

There are many benefits to using Gua Sha for lower back pain, including:

Reducing pain and tension - Gua Sha can help to reduce pain and tension in the lower back, promoting relaxation and reducing discomfort.

Improving circulation - Gua Sha can improve circulation in the lower back, promoting healing and reducing inflammation.

Reducing inflammation - Gua Sha can help to reduce inflammation in the lower back, which can contribute to pain and discomfort.

Promoting relaxation - Gua Sha is a holistic technique that can promote overall well-being and relaxation, reducing stress and tension in the body.

Gua Sha Techniques for Lower Back Pain

Some of the Gua Sha techniques used for lower back pain include:

Lower Back - Use the Gua Sha tool to scrape the lower back in an upward motion towards the waist, focusing on areas where tension and discomfort are present.

Glutes - Use the Gua Sha tool to scrape the glutes in an upward motion towards the waist, focusing on areas where tension and discomfort are present.

IT Band - Use the Gua Sha tool to scrape the IT band in a downward motion towards the knee, focusing on areas where tension and discomfort are present.

Quadratus Lumborum - Use the Gua Sha tool to scrape the quadratus lumborum muscle, which is located on the side of the lower back, focusing on areas where tension and discomfort are present.

It is important to note that Gua Sha for lower back pain should be performed by a trained and qualified practitioner, or under their guidance. The technique should be performed gently and without causing pain or discomfort to the individual.

## Improving hip mobility

Hip mobility is an important aspect of overall mobility and movement in the body. The hips are involved in many daily activities, such as walking, running, and sitting, and when they are not functioning properly, it can lead to pain and discomfort. Gua Sha is a traditional Chinese medicine technique that can be used to improve hip mobility. Below we will explore how Gua Sha can be used to improve hip mobility.

What is Gua Sha?

Gua Sha is a traditional Chinese medicine technique that involves using a smooth-edged tool to scrape the skin in a firm and repetitive manner. The technique is used to stimulate the flow of energy, or Qi, throughout the body, and it is often used to promote relaxation, relieve pain, and improve circulation.

How Does Gua Sha Work for Hip Mobility?

Gua Sha for hip mobility involves using the Gua Sha tool to apply pressure and scraping motions to specific points on the hips. These points are located along the meridian lines of the body, which are the energy channels that run throughout the body. By stimulating these points, Gua Sha can promote the flow of energy and reduce tension in the hip muscles, leading to improved mobility.

Benefits of Gua Sha for Hip Mobility

There are many benefits to using Gua Sha for hip mobility, including:

Improving range of motion - Gua Sha can help to improve the range of motion in the hips, promoting better mobility and movement.

Reducing pain and tension - Gua Sha can help to reduce pain and tension in the hip muscles, promoting relaxation and reducing discomfort.

Improving circulation - Gua Sha can improve circulation in the hips, promoting healing and reducing inflammation.

Promoting relaxation - Gua Sha is a holistic technique that can promote overall well-being and relaxation, reducing stress and tension in the body.

Gua Sha Techniques for Hip Mobility

Some of the Gua Sha techniques used for hip mobility include:

Hip Flexors - Use the Gua Sha tool to scrape the hip flexors, which are located at the front of the hips, focusing on areas where tension and discomfort are present.

Glutes - Use the Gua Sha tool to scrape the glutes, which are located at the back of the hips, focusing on areas where tension and discomfort are present.

IT Band - Use the Gua Sha tool to scrape the IT band, which runs along the outside of the hip, focusing on areas where tension and discomfort are present.

Piriformis - Use the Gua Sha tool to scrape the piriformis muscle, which is located deep in the hip, focusing on areas where tension and discomfort are present.

It is important to note that Gua Sha for hip mobility should be performed by a trained and qualified practitioner, or under their guidance. The technique should be performed gently and without causing pain or discomfort to the individual.

Chapter Nine

# Gua Sha for the Arms and Hands

Gua Sha is a traditional Chinese medicine technique that involves using a smooth-edged tool to scrape the skin in a firm and repetitive manner. The technique is used to stimulate the flow of energy, or Qi, throughout the body, and it is often used to promote relaxation, relieve pain, and improve circulation. Below we will explore how Gua Sha can be used to promote arm and hand health.

Why Is Arm and Hand Health Important?

Arm and hand health is important because they are used in many daily activities such as typing, writing, and carrying objects. When arm and hand muscles become tight or tense, it can lead to pain and discomfort, making it difficult to perform these activities. Additionally, tight muscles can lead to reduced range of motion and decreased mobility in the arms and hands.

How Does Gua Sha Work for Arms and Hands?

Gua Sha for arms and hands involves using the Gua Sha tool to apply pressure and scraping motions to specific points on the arms and hands. These points are located along the meridian lines of the body, which are the energy channels that run throughout the body. By stimulating these points, Gua Sha can promote the flow of energy and reduce tension in the arm and hand muscles, leading to improved mobility and reduced pain and discomfort.

Benefits of Gua Sha for Arms and Hands

There are many benefits to using Gua Sha for arms and hands, including:

Reducing pain and tension - Gua Sha can help to reduce pain and tension in the arm and hand muscles, promoting relaxation and reducing discomfort.

Improving circulation - Gua Sha can improve circulation in the arms and hands, promoting healing and reducing inflammation.

Improving range of motion - Gua Sha can help to improve the range of motion in the arms and hands, promoting better mobility and movement.

Promoting relaxation - Gua Sha is a holistic technique that can promote overall well-being and relaxation, reducing stress and tension in the body.

Gua Sha Techniques for Arms and Hands

Some of the Gua Sha techniques used for arms and hands include:

Forearms - Use the Gua Sha tool to scrape the forearms, focusing on areas where tension and discomfort are present.

Wrist - Use the Gua Sha tool to scrape the wrist, focusing on areas where tension and discomfort are present.

Hands - Use the Gua Sha tool to scrape the hands, focusing on areas where tension and discomfort are present.

It is important to note that Gua Sha for arms and hands should be performed by a trained and qualified practitioner, or under their guidance. The technique should be performed gently and without causing pain or discomfort to the individual.

## Carpal tunnel relief

Carpal tunnel syndrome is a common condition that affects many people, particularly those who perform repetitive hand motions or work at a desk for long periods of time. It is caused by the compression of the median nerve in the wrist, leading to pain, tingling, and numbness in the hand and fingers. Gua Sha is a traditional Chinese medicine technique that can be used to alleviate symptoms of carpal tunnel syndrome. Below we will explore how Gua Sha can be used for carpal tunnel relief.

What is Carpal Tunnel Syndrome?

Carpal tunnel syndrome is a condition that occurs when the median nerve in the wrist becomes compressed, causing pain, tingling, and numbness in the hand and fingers. The condition can be caused by repetitive hand motions, such as typing or using a mouse, or by certain medical conditions such as diabetes or hypothyroidism.

How Does Gua Sha Work for Carpal Tunnel Relief?

Gua Sha for carpal tunnel relief involves using the Gua Sha tool to apply pressure and scraping motions to specific points on the wrist and hand. These points are located along the meridian lines of the body, which are the energy channels that run throughout the body. By stimulating these points, Gua Sha can promote the flow of energy and reduce tension in the wrist and hand muscles, leading to improved mobility and reduced pain and discomfort.

Benefits of Gua Sha for Carpal Tunnel Relief

There are many benefits to using Gua Sha for carpal tunnel relief, including:

Reducing pain and discomfort - Gua Sha can help to reduce pain and discomfort in the wrist and hand, making it easier to perform daily activities.

Improving circulation - Gua Sha can improve circulation in the wrist and hand, promoting healing and reducing inflammation.

Promoting relaxation - Gua Sha is a holistic technique that can promote overall well-being and relaxation, reducing stress and tension in the body.

Improving mobility - Gua Sha can help to improve the range of motion in the wrist and hand, promoting better movement and reducing stiffness.

Gua Sha Techniques for Carpal Tunnel Relief

Some of the Gua Sha techniques used for carpal tunnel relief include:

Wrist - Use the Gua Sha tool to scrape the wrist, focusing on areas where tension and discomfort are present.

Forearm - Use the Gua Sha tool to scrape the forearm, focusing on areas where tension and discomfort are present.

Hand - Use the Gua Sha tool to scrape the hand, focusing on areas where tension and discomfort are present.

It is important to note that Gua Sha for carpal tunnel relief should be performed by a trained and qualified practitioner, or under their guidance. The technique should be performed gently and without causing pain or discomfort to the individual.

## Increasing circulation

Increasing circulation is essential for maintaining good health and promoting healing throughout the body. Poor circulation can lead to a variety of health problems, including muscle and joint pain, numbness, and tingling. Gua Sha is a traditional Chinese medicine technique that can help to increase circulation and promote overall well-being. Below we will explore how Gua Sha can be used to increase circulation.

What is Circulation?

Circulation refers to the movement of blood throughout the body. Blood carries oxygen and nutrients to the cells, tissues, and organs of the body, and removes waste and carbon dioxide. Good circulation is essential for maintaining optimal health, as it helps to promote healing and repair throughout the body.

How Does Gua Sha Work for Increasing Circulation?

Gua Sha works by stimulating the flow of energy, or Qi, throughout the body. The technique involves using a smooth-edged tool to scrape the skin in a firm and repetitive manner, which can help to release tension and promote the movement of energy and blood.

Benefits of Gua Sha for Increasing Circulation

There are many benefits to using Gua Sha for increasing circulation, including:

Improving oxygen flow - Gua Sha can improve the flow of oxygen-rich blood to the cells, promoting healing and repair.

Reducing inflammation - Gua Sha can reduce inflammation by improving circulation and promoting the movement of lymphatic fluid.

Reducing pain - Gua Sha can help to reduce pain by increasing circulation and promoting the release of endorphins, the body's natural painkillers.

Promoting relaxation - Gua Sha is a holistic technique that can promote relaxation and reduce stress, leading to improved overall well-being.

Gua Sha Techniques for Increasing Circulation

Some of the Gua Sha techniques used for increasing circulation include:

Back - Use the Gua Sha tool to scrape the back, focusing on areas where tension and discomfort are present.

Legs - Use the Gua Sha tool to scrape the legs, focusing on areas where tension and discomfort are present.

Arms - Use the Gua Sha tool to scrape the arms, focusing on areas where tension and discomfort are present.

It is important to note that Gua Sha should be performed by a trained and qualified practitioner, or under their guidance. The technique should be performed gently and without causing pain or discomfort to the individual.

Chapter Ten

# Gua Sha for the Legs and Feet

Gua Sha is a traditional Chinese medicine technique that has been used for thousands of years to promote healing and improve overall well-being. This technique involves using a smooth-edged tool to scrape the skin in a firm and repetitive manner, which can help to release tension and promote the movement of energy and blood. Gua Sha can be used to treat a variety of health conditions, including those related to the legs and feet. Below we will explore how Gua Sha can be used for the legs and feet.

Gua Sha Techniques for the Legs and Feet

Some of the Gua Sha techniques used for the legs and feet include:

Calves - Use the Gua Sha tool to scrape the calves, focusing on areas where tension and discomfort are present.

Thighs - Use the Gua Sha tool to scrape the thighs, focusing on areas where tension and discomfort are present.

Feet - Use the Gua Sha tool to scrape the feet, focusing on areas where tension and discomfort are present.

Benefits of Gua Sha for the Legs and Feet

There are many benefits to using Gua Sha for the legs and feet, including:

Reducing pain and discomfort - Gua Sha can help to reduce pain and discomfort in the legs and feet, making it easier to perform daily activities.

Improving circulation - Gua Sha can improve circulation in the legs and feet, promoting healing and reducing inflammation.

Promoting relaxation - Gua Sha is a holistic technique that can promote overall well-being and relaxation, reducing stress and tension in the body.

Improving mobility - Gua Sha can help to improve the range of motion in the legs and feet, promoting better movement and reducing stiffness.

Alleviating swelling - Gua Sha can help to alleviate swelling in the legs and feet by promoting the movement of lymphatic fluid.

Gua Sha for Leg and Foot Conditions

Gua Sha can be used to treat a variety of leg and foot conditions, including:

Plantar fasciitis - Gua Sha can help to reduce pain and inflammation in the plantar fascia, which is the band of tissue that runs along the bottom of the foot.

Shin splints - Gua Sha can help to reduce pain and inflammation in the shins, which can be caused by overuse or improper footwear.

Ankle sprains - Gua Sha can help to reduce pain and inflammation in the ankle, promoting healing and reducing stiffness.

Leg cramps - Gua Sha can help to reduce tension in the muscles of the legs, promoting relaxation and reducing the likelihood of leg cramps.

It is important to note that Gua Sha should be performed by a trained and qualified practitioner, or under their guidance. The technique should be performed gently and without causing pain or discomfort to the individual.

## Reducing leg cramps

Leg cramps are a common problem that can be caused by a variety of factors, including dehydration, muscle fatigue, and poor circulation. Leg cramps can be painful and disruptive to daily activities, making it important to find effective treatment options. Gua Sha is a traditional Chinese medicine technique that has been used for thousands of years to promote healing and improve overall well-being. Below we will explore how Gua Sha can be used to reduce leg cramps.

What are Leg Cramps?

Leg cramps are a sudden and involuntary contraction of the muscles in the leg. They can occur at any time, but are most commonly experienced at night or during periods of physical activity. Leg cramps can be caused by a variety of factors, including dehydration, muscle fatigue, and poor circulation.

How Does Gua Sha Work for Reducing Leg Cramps?

Gua Sha works by stimulating the flow of energy, or Qi, throughout the body. The technique involves using a smooth-edged tool to scrape the skin in a firm and repetitive manner, which can help to release tension and promote the movement of energy and blood. By promoting circulation and releasing tension in the muscles, Gua Sha can help to reduce the likelihood of leg cramps.

Benefits of Gua Sha for Reducing Leg Cramps

There are many benefits to using Gua Sha for reducing leg cramps, including:

Promoting relaxation - Gua Sha is a holistic technique that can promote relaxation and reduce stress, which can contribute to the onset of leg cramps.

Improving circulation - Gua Sha can improve circulation in the legs, promoting healing and reducing the likelihood of leg cramps.

Reducing tension - Gua Sha can help to release tension in the muscles, reducing the likelihood of muscle cramps.

Gua Sha Techniques for Reducing Leg Cramps

Some of the Gua Sha techniques used for reducing leg cramps include:

Calves - Use the Gua Sha tool to scrape the calves, focusing on areas where tension and discomfort are present.

Thighs - Use the Gua Sha tool to scrape the thighs, focusing on areas where tension and discomfort are present.

Feet - Use the Gua Sha tool to scrape the feet, focusing on areas where tension and discomfort are present.

It is important to note that Gua Sha should be performed by a trained and qualified practitioner, or under their guidance. The technique should be performed gently and without causing pain or discomfort to the individual.

## Foot and ankle pain relief

Foot and ankle pain is a common problem that affects millions of people worldwide. This type of pain can be caused by a variety of factors, including injuries, overuse, and medical conditions like arthritis. Foot and ankle pain can be debilitating and interfere with daily activities, making it important to find effective treatment options. Gua Sha is a traditional Chinese medicine technique that has been used for thousands of years to promote healing and improve overall well-being. Below we will explore how Gua Sha can be used to relieve foot and ankle pain.

What Causes Foot and Ankle Pain?

Foot and ankle pain can be caused by a variety of factors, including:

Injuries - Sprains, strains, and fractures can all cause foot and ankle pain.

Overuse - Activities that involve repetitive motions, like running or dancing, can cause foot and ankle pain.

Medical conditions - Medical conditions like arthritis, plantar fasciitis, and gout can all cause foot and ankle pain.

How Does Gua Sha Work for Foot and Ankle Pain Relief?

Gua Sha works by stimulating the flow of energy, or Qi, throughout the body. The technique involves using a smooth-edged tool to scrape the skin in a firm and repetitive manner, which can help to release tension and promote the movement of energy and blood. By promoting circulation and releasing tension in the muscles, Gua Sha can help to reduce foot and ankle pain.

Benefits of Gua Sha for Foot and Ankle Pain Relief

There are many benefits to using Gua Sha for foot and ankle pain relief, including:

Pain relief - Gua Sha can help to reduce pain in the feet and ankles by releasing tension and promoting circulation.

Improved range of motion - Gua Sha can help to improve range of motion in the feet and ankles by reducing stiffness and promoting flexibility.

Stress reduction - Gua Sha is a holistic technique that can promote relaxation and reduce stress, which can contribute to foot and ankle pain.

Gua Sha Techniques for Foot and Ankle Pain Relief

Some of the Gua Sha techniques used for foot and ankle pain relief include:

Ankle - Use the Gua Sha tool to scrape the ankle, focusing on areas where tension and discomfort are present.

Arch of the foot - Use the Gua Sha tool to scrape the arch of the foot, focusing on areas where tension and discomfort are present.

Heel - Use the Gua Sha tool to scrape the heel, focusing on areas where tension and discomfort are present.

It is important to note that Gua Sha should be performed by a trained and qualified practitioner, or under their guidance. The technique should be performed gently and without causing pain or discomfort to the individual.

Chapter Eleven

# Gua Sha for Stress Relief

Stress is a common problem that affects millions of people worldwide. Stress can be caused by a variety of factors, including work, relationships, finances, and health issues. Chronic stress can lead to a range of physical and mental health problems, including anxiety, depression, and insomnia. Gua Sha is a traditional Chinese medicine technique that has been used for thousands of years to promote healing and improve overall well-being. Below we will explore how Gua Sha can be used for stress relief.

What is Gua Sha?

Gua Sha is a technique used in traditional Chinese medicine that involves using a smooth-edged tool to scrape the skin in a firm and repetitive manner. The technique is designed to stimulate the flow of energy, or Qi, throughout the body. By promoting circulation and releasing tension in the muscles, Gua Sha can help to promote healing and improve overall well-being.

Benefits of Gua Sha for Stress Relief

There are many benefits to using Gua Sha for stress relief, including:

Relaxation - Gua Sha is a holistic technique that can promote relaxation and reduce stress.

Improved mood - Gua Sha can help to improve mood by reducing stress and promoting feelings of well-being.

Improved sleep - Gua Sha can help to improve sleep by reducing stress and promoting relaxation.

Gua Sha Techniques for Stress Relief

Some of the Gua Sha techniques used for stress relief include:

Neck - Use the Gua Sha tool to scrape the neck, focusing on areas where tension and discomfort are present.

Shoulders - Use the Gua Sha tool to scrape the shoulders, focusing on areas where tension and discomfort are present.

Back - Use the Gua Sha tool to scrape the back, focusing on areas where tension and discomfort are present.

It is important to note that Gua Sha should be performed by a trained and qualified practitioner, or under their guidance. The technique should be performed gently and without causing pain or discomfort to the individual.

Gua Sha Oils for Stress Relief

Gua Sha can be performed using a variety of oils, which can help to enhance the relaxation and stress-relieving benefits of the technique. Some of the most popular oils used for Gua Sha include:

Lavender oil - Lavender oil is known for its calming and soothing properties, which can help to promote relaxation and reduce stress.

Peppermint oil - Peppermint oil is known for its invigorating and energizing properties, which can help to reduce stress and promote feelings of well-being.

Eucalyptus oil - Eucalyptus oil is known for its calming and soothing properties, which can help to promote relaxation and reduce stress.

Preparing for a Gua Sha Session for Stress Relief

To prepare for a Gua Sha session for stress relief, it is important to create a comfortable and relaxing environment. Some tips for creating a relaxing environment include:

Choosing a quiet and peaceful space to perform the technique.

Using soft lighting, such as candles or dimmed lamps.

Playing calming music or nature sounds.

Using a comfortable and supportive surface to lie on, such as a yoga mat or massage table.

## Relaxation techniques

Relaxation techniques are important tools that can help individuals reduce stress and promote a sense of calm and well-being. With the many stressors that we face in our daily lives, finding effective relaxation techniques can be crucial for maintaining physical and mental health. Gua Sha is a traditional Chinese medicine technique that has been used for thousands of years to promote relaxation and improve overall well-being. Below we will explore how Gua Sha can be used as a relaxation technique.

What is Gua Sha?

Gua Sha is a technique used in traditional Chinese medicine that involves using a smooth-edged tool to scrape the skin in a firm and repetitive manner. The technique is designed to stimulate the flow of energy, or Qi, throughout the body. By promoting circulation and releasing tension in the muscles, Gua Sha can help to promote healing and improve overall well-being.

Benefits of Gua Sha as a Relaxation Technique

There are many benefits to using Gua Sha as a relaxation technique, including:

Reduced muscle tension - Gua Sha can help to release tension in the muscles, promoting relaxation and reducing feelings of tightness and discomfort.

Improved circulation - By promoting circulation, Gua Sha can help to improve the flow of oxygen and nutrients throughout the body, which can promote relaxation and reduce feelings of stress.

Promotes a sense of calm - Gua Sha is a gentle and soothing technique that can promote a sense of calm and relaxation.

Gua Sha Techniques for Relaxation

Some of the Gua Sha techniques used for relaxation include:

Neck - Use the Gua Sha tool to scrape the neck, focusing on areas where tension and discomfort are present.

Shoulders - Use the Gua Sha tool to scrape the shoulders, focusing on areas where tension and discomfort are present.

Back - Use the Gua Sha tool to scrape the back, focusing on areas where tension and discomfort are present.

It is important to note that Gua Sha should be performed by a trained and qualified practitioner, or under their guidance. The technique should be performed gently and without causing pain or discomfort to the individual.

Gua Sha Oils for Relaxation

Gua Sha can be performed using a variety of oils, which can help to enhance the relaxation and stress-relieving benefits of the technique. Some of the most popular oils used for Gua Sha include:

Lavender oil - Lavender oil is known for its calming and soothing properties, which can help to promote relaxation and reduce stress.

Peppermint oil - Peppermint oil is known for its invigorating and energizing properties, which can help to reduce stress and promote feelings of well-being.

Eucalyptus oil - Eucalyptus oil is known for its calming and soothing properties, which can help to promote relaxation and reduce stress.

Preparing for a Gua Sha Session for Relaxation

To prepare for a Gua Sha session for relaxation, it is important to create a comfortable and relaxing environment. Some tips for creating a relaxing environment include:

Choosing a quiet and peaceful space to perform the technique.

Using soft lighting, such as candles or dimmed lamps.

Playing calming music or nature sounds.

Using a comfortable and supportive surface to lie on, such as a yoga mat or massage table.

## Balancing the nervous system

The nervous system is a complex network of cells and tissues that is responsible for regulating and coordinating the functions of the body. When the nervous system is imbalanced, it can lead to a variety of physical and mental health problems, including anxiety, depression, and chronic pain. Gua Sha is a traditional Chinese medicine technique that has been used for centuries to help balance the nervous system and promote overall health and well-being. Below we will explore how Gua Sha can be used to balance the nervous system.

What is Gua Sha?

Gua Sha is a technique that involves scraping the skin with a smooth-edged tool to promote healing and balance in the body. The technique is used in traditional Chinese medicine to stimulate the flow of energy, or Qi, throughout the body. By promoting circulation and releasing tension in the muscles, Gua Sha can help to promote healing and improve overall well-being.

Benefits of Gua Sha for Balancing the Nervous System

There are many benefits to using Gua Sha for balancing the nervous system, including:

Reduced stress and anxiety - Gua Sha can help to reduce stress and anxiety by promoting relaxation and reducing tension in the muscles.

Improved circulation - Gua Sha can help to improve circulation, which can help to promote the delivery of oxygen and nutrients to the cells of the body, including the nervous system.

Promotes a sense of calm - Gua Sha is a gentle and soothing technique that can promote a sense of calm and relaxation, which can help to reduce feelings of anxiety and stress.

## Gua Sha Techniques for Balancing the Nervous System

Some of the Gua Sha techniques used for balancing the nervous system include:

Neck - Use the Gua Sha tool to scrape the neck, focusing on areas where tension and discomfort are present. This can help to promote relaxation and reduce feelings of anxiety and stress.

Head - Use the Gua Sha tool to scrape the head, focusing on areas where tension and discomfort are present. This can help to promote relaxation and reduce feelings of anxiety and stress.

Back - Use the Gua Sha tool to scrape the back, focusing on areas where tension and discomfort are present. This can help to promote relaxation and reduce feelings of anxiety and stress.

It is important to note that Gua Sha should be performed by a trained and qualified practitioner, or under their guidance. The technique should be performed gently and without causing pain or discomfort to the individual.

## Gua Sha Oils for Balancing the Nervous System

Gua Sha can be performed using a variety of oils, which can help to enhance the balancing and stress-relieving benefits of the technique. Some of the most popular oils used for Gua Sha include:

Lavender oil - Lavender oil is known for its calming and soothing properties, which can help to promote relaxation and reduce stress and anxiety.

Frankincense oil - Frankincense oil is known for its grounding and balancing properties, which can help to promote a sense of calm and well-being.

Rose oil - Rose oil is known for its ability to promote relaxation and reduce feelings of stress and anxiety.

Preparing for a Gua Sha Session for Balancing the Nervous System

To prepare for a Gua Sha session for balancing the nervous system, it is important to create a calm and relaxing environment. Some tips for creating a relaxing environment include:

Choosing a quiet and peaceful space to perform the technique.

Using soft lighting, such as candles or dimmed lamps.

Playing calming music or nature sounds.

Using a comfortable and supportive surface to lie on, such as a yoga mat or massage table.

Chapter Twelve

# Gua Sha for Boosting Immunity

The immune system is responsible for protecting the body against viruses, bacteria, and other harmful substances. When the immune system is weakened, it can lead to a variety of health problems, including frequent colds and infections. Gua Sha is a traditional Chinese medicine technique that has been used for centuries to promote health and well-being. In recent years, there has been growing interest in the use of Gua Sha for boosting immunity. Below we will explore how Gua Sha can be used to boost immunity.

What is Gua Sha?

Gua Sha is a technique that involves scraping the skin with a smooth-edged tool to promote healing and balance in the body. The technique is used in traditional Chinese medicine to stimulate the flow of energy, or Qi, throughout the body. By promoting circulation and releasing tension in the muscles, Gua Sha can help to promote healing and improve overall well-being.

Benefits of Gua Sha for Boosting Immunity

There are many benefits to using Gua Sha for boosting immunity, including:

Improved circulation - Gua Sha can help to improve circulation, which can help to promote the delivery of oxygen and nutrients to the cells of the body, including the immune system.

Increased lymphatic flow - Gua Sha can help to increase lymphatic flow, which is responsible for removing waste and toxins from the body. This can help to support the immune system by removing harmful substances.

Reduced inflammation - Gua Sha can help to reduce inflammation, which can be a contributing factor to a weakened immune system.

Gua Sha Techniques for Boosting Immunity

Some of the Gua Sha techniques used for boosting immunity include:

Chest and back - Use the Gua Sha tool to scrape the chest and back, focusing on areas where tension and discomfort are present. This can help to promote circulation and lymphatic flow in the area.

Neck - Use the Gua Sha tool to scrape the neck, focusing on areas where tension and discomfort are present. This can help to promote circulation and lymphatic flow in the area.

Arms and legs - Use the Gua Sha tool to scrape the arms and legs, focusing on areas where tension and discomfort are present. This can help to promote circulation and lymphatic flow in the area.

It is important to note that Gua Sha should be performed by a trained and qualified practitioner, or under their guidance. The technique should be performed gently and without causing pain or discomfort to the individual.

Gua Sha Oils for Boosting Immunity

Gua Sha can be performed using a variety of oils, which can help to enhance the immune-boosting benefits of the technique. Some of the most popular oils used for Gua Sha include:

Eucalyptus oil - Eucalyptus oil is known for its antibacterial and antiviral properties, which can help to support the immune system.

Tea tree oil - Tea tree oil is known for its antimicrobial properties, which can help to fight off harmful bacteria and viruses.

Peppermint oil - Peppermint oil is known for its ability to promote circulation and stimulate the immune system.

Preparing for a Gua Sha Session for Boosting Immunity

To prepare for a Gua Sha session for boosting immunity, it is important to create a calm and relaxing environment. Some tips for creating a relaxing environment include:

Choosing a quiet and peaceful space to perform the technique.

Using soft lighting, such as candles or dimmed lamps.

Playing calming music or nature sounds.

Using a comfortable and supportive surface to lie on, such as a yoga mat or massage table.

## Stimulating the immune system

The immune system is responsible for protecting the body against harmful substances such as viruses, bacteria, and toxins. A healthy immune system is essential for overall health and well-being. There are many ways to support the immune system, including diet, exercise, and stress reduction techniques. In recent years, Gua Sha, a traditional Chinese medicine technique, has gained popularity as a way to stimulate the immune system. Below we will explore how Gua Sha can stimulate the immune system and promote overall health.

What is Gua Sha?

Gua Sha is a traditional Chinese medicine technique that involves scraping the skin with a smooth-edged tool. The goal of Gua Sha is to stimulate the flow of energy, or Qi, throughout the body. By promoting circulation and releasing tension in the muscles, Gua Sha can help to promote healing and improve overall well-being.

How Does Gua Sha Stimulate the Immune System?

There are many ways in which Gua Sha can stimulate the immune system, including:

Promoting circulation - Gua Sha can help to promote circulation throughout the body, including the lymphatic system. This can help to improve the flow of immune cells and other nutrients throughout the body, leading to improved immune function.

Reducing inflammation - Gua Sha can help to reduce inflammation, which can be a contributing factor to a weakened immune system. By reducing inflammation, Gua Sha can help to support a healthy immune response.

Supporting the lymphatic system - The lymphatic system is responsible for removing waste and toxins from the body. Gua Sha can help to support lymphatic flow, which can help to remove harmful substances from the body and support the immune system.

Gua Sha Techniques for Stimulating the Immune System

Some of the Gua Sha techniques used for stimulating the immune system include:

Chest and back - Use the Gua Sha tool to scrape the chest and back, focusing on areas where tension and discomfort are present. This can help to promote circulation and lymphatic flow in the area.

Neck - Use the Gua Sha tool to scrape the neck, focusing on areas where tension and discomfort are present. This can help to promote circulation and lymphatic flow in the area.

Arms and legs - Use the Gua Sha tool to scrape the arms and legs, focusing on areas where tension and discomfort are present. This can help to promote circulation and lymphatic flow in the area.

It is important to note that Gua Sha should be performed by a trained and qualified practitioner, or under their guidance. The technique should be performed gently and without causing pain or discomfort to the individual.

Gua Sha Oils for Stimulating the Immune System

Gua Sha can be performed using a variety of oils, which can help to enhance the immune-boosting benefits of the technique. Some of the most popular oils used for Gua Sha include:

Eucalyptus oil - Eucalyptus oil is known for its antibacterial and antiviral properties, which can help to support the immune system.

Tea tree oil - Tea tree oil is known for its antimicrobial properties, which can help to fight off harmful bacteria and viruses.

Peppermint oil - Peppermint oil is known for its ability to promote circulation and stimulate the immune system.

Preparing for a Gua Sha Session for Immune Stimulation

To prepare for a Gua Sha session for immune stimulation, it is important to create a calm and relaxing environment. Some tips for creating a relaxing environment include:

Choosing a quiet and peaceful space to perform the technique.

Using soft lighting, such as candles or dimmed lamps.

Playing calming music or nature sounds.

Using a comfortable and supportive surface to lie

## Lymphatic drainage

The lymphatic system is responsible for removing waste and toxins from the body, and is an important part of the immune system. Lymphatic drainage is a technique used to help support the lymphatic system and promote overall health. Gua Sha, a traditional Chinese medicine technique, can be used to support lymphatic drainage and promote a healthy immune system. Below we will explore the benefits of lymphatic drainage and how Gua Sha can be used to support lymphatic drainage.

What is Lymphatic Drainage?

Lymphatic drainage is a technique used to promote the movement of lymphatic fluid throughout the body. The lymphatic system is responsible for removing waste and toxins from the body, and supporting the immune system. When the lymphatic system becomes congested or sluggish, it can lead to a variety of health problems, including swelling, inflammation, and a weakened immune system.

Lymphatic drainage techniques can be used to help promote the movement of lymphatic fluid, which can help to support overall health and well-being. These techniques can include massage, dry brushing, and Gua Sha.

How Does Gua Sha Support Lymphatic Drainage?

Gua Sha is a technique that involves scraping the skin with a smooth-edged tool. The goal of Gua Sha is to promote circulation, release tension in the muscles, and stimulate the flow of energy, or Qi, throughout the body. By promoting circulation and lymphatic flow, Gua Sha can help to support lymphatic drainage and promote overall health.

There are several ways in which Gua Sha can support lymphatic drainage, including:

Promoting circulation - Gua Sha can help to promote circulation throughout the body, including the lymphatic system. This can help to improve the flow of lymphatic fluid and other nutrients throughout the body, leading to improved immune function.

Reducing inflammation - Gua Sha can help to reduce inflammation, which can be a contributing factor to lymphatic congestion. By reducing inflammation, Gua Sha can help to support the movement of lymphatic fluid.

Releasing tension - Gua Sha can help to release tension in the muscles, which can be a contributing factor to lymphatic congestion. By releasing tension, Gua Sha can help to support lymphatic flow and promote overall health.

Gua Sha Techniques for Supporting Lymphatic Drainage

Some of the Gua Sha techniques used for supporting lymphatic drainage include:

Face and neck - Use the Gua Sha tool to gently scrape the face and neck, focusing on areas where tension and discomfort are present. This can help to promote lymphatic flow in the area.

Arms and legs - Use the Gua Sha tool to gently scrape the arms and legs, focusing on areas where tension and discomfort are present. This can help to promote lymphatic flow in the area.

Back and shoulders - Use the Gua Sha tool to gently scrape the back and shoulders, focusing on areas where tension and discomfort are present. This can help to promote lymphatic flow in the area.

It is important to note that Gua Sha should be performed by a trained and qualified practitioner, or under their guidance. The technique should be performed gently and without causing pain or discomfort to the individual.

Gua Sha Oils for Supporting Lymphatic Drainage

Gua Sha can be performed using a variety of oils, which can help to enhance the lymphatic drainage benefits of the technique. Some of the most popular oils used for Gua Sha include:

Ginger oil - Ginger oil is known for its ability to promote circulation and stimulate the lymphatic system.

Cypress oil - Cypress oil is known for its ability to promote lymphatic flow and reduce inflammation.

Rosemary oil - Rosemary oil is known for its ability to stimulate circulation

Chapter Thirteen

# Gua Sha for Digestive Health

Gua Sha, a traditional Chinese medicine technique, has been used for centuries to promote digestive health. This therapy involves scraping the skin using a smooth-edged tool, which helps to stimulate blood flow and lymphatic drainage in the body. By doing so, Gua Sha can help relieve digestive symptoms such as bloating, constipation, and abdominal discomfort.

One of the ways that Gua Sha can improve digestive health is by increasing circulation in the digestive organs. This technique helps to bring fresh blood and nutrients to the area, which can promote healing and relieve inflammation. It can also stimulate the movement of the digestive muscles, helping to alleviate constipation and bloating.

In addition, Gua Sha can help to stimulate the lymphatic system, which is responsible for removing waste and toxins from the body. By doing so, this technique can help to improve overall digestion and reduce the risk of gastrointestinal issues.

When performing Gua Sha for digestive health, the practitioner will typically target the stomach, intestines, and other digestive organs. They may use different strokes and techniques to address specific digestive concerns, such as using a circular motion to target bloating or a back-and-forth motion to address constipation.

Some common lubricants used during Gua Sha for digestive health include ginger oil and peppermint oil. These oils have natural anti-inflammatory properties and can help to soothe the digestive tract. They can also enhance the effects of Gua Sha by increasing blood flow and promoting relaxation.

It is important to note that while Gua Sha can be a beneficial therapy for digestive health, it should not be used as a substitute for medical treatment. If you are experiencing severe digestive symptoms, it is important to consult with a healthcare professional before beginning any new therapy.

In addition, it is important to seek out a qualified and experienced practitioner when receiving Gua Sha therapy. Improper use of Gua Sha tools or techniques can lead to injury or other complications.

## Improving digestion

Digestive problems such as bloating, constipation, and indigestion can have a significant impact on our daily lives. While there are various treatments available, some people are turning to traditional Chinese medicine techniques such as Gua Sha to improve their digestive health. Below we will explore how Gua Sha can help to improve digestion and alleviate common digestive symptoms.

Gua Sha is a form of traditional Chinese medicine that involves scraping the skin using a smooth-edged tool. This technique has been used for centuries to promote healing and improve overall well-being. Gua Sha works by stimulating blood flow and promoting lymphatic drainage in the body, which can help to relieve inflammation and promote healing.

One way that Gua Sha can improve digestion is by promoting blood flow to the digestive organs. When blood flow is increased, the organs receive more oxygen and nutrients, which can help to promote healing and reduce inflammation. In addition, Gua Sha can stimulate the movement of the digestive muscles, helping to relieve constipation and bloating.

Another way that Gua Sha can improve digestion is by promoting lymphatic drainage. The lymphatic system is responsible for removing waste and toxins from the body. When the lymphatic system is functioning properly, it can help to improve overall digestion and reduce the risk of gastrointestinal issues.

Gua Sha can be performed on various parts of the body to improve digestion. For example, the stomach, intestines, and other digestive organs can be targeted to alleviate digestive symptoms. The practitioner may use different strokes and techniques depending on the specific digestive concerns.

Ginger oil and peppermint oil are two common lubricants used during Gua Sha for digestive health. These oils have natural anti-inflammatory properties and can help to soothe the digestive tract. They can also enhance the effects of Gua Sha by increasing blood flow and promoting relaxation.

In addition to Gua Sha, there are other traditional Chinese medicine techniques that can help to improve digestion. Acupuncture, for example, can help to stimulate the digestive system and promote healing. Herbal remedies such as ginger, turmeric, and fennel can also be used to alleviate digestive symptoms.

It is important to note that while Gua Sha and other traditional Chinese medicine techniques can be beneficial for improving digestion, they should not be used as a substitute for medical treatment. If you are experiencing severe digestive symptoms, it is important to consult with a healthcare professional before beginning any new therapy.

In addition, it is important to seek out a qualified and experienced practitioner when receiving Gua Sha therapy. Improper use of Gua Sha tools or techniques can lead to injury or other complications.

## Alleviating constipation

Gua Sha is a traditional Chinese medicine technique that involves scraping the skin to stimulate circulation, relieve tension, and promote healing. It has been used for thousands of years to treat a wide range of conditions, including digestive issues such as constipation.

Constipation is a common digestive problem that affects millions of people worldwide. It is characterized by infrequent bowel movements, difficulty passing stools, and abdominal discomfort. While there are many causes of constipation, including poor diet, dehydration, and lack of physical activity, it is often a symptom of an underlying health condition, such as irritable bowel syndrome or colon cancer.

Gua Sha can be an effective natural remedy for constipation, as it helps to stimulate the digestive system and promote bowel movements. The technique works by applying pressure to specific points on the abdomen and back, which helps to release tension and improve circulation in the digestive organs.

To perform Gua Sha for constipation, you will need a Gua Sha tool, such as a flat stone or ceramic plate, as well as a lubricant, such as oil or lotion. Begin by applying a small amount of lubricant to the abdomen and lower back, then use the Gua Sha tool to gently scrape the skin in a downward motion, starting from the ribcage and moving towards the pubic bone.

Focus on the areas where you feel the most tension or discomfort, applying moderate pressure and gradually increasing the intensity as you go. You may also want to use circular or zig-zag strokes to target specific areas of the digestive system, such as the colon or small intestine.

Repeat this process for several minutes, taking breaks as needed to avoid causing discomfort or irritation. It is important to listen to your body and adjust the pressure and intensity of the strokes as necessary to ensure a comfortable and effective treatment.

In addition to Gua Sha, there are several other natural remedies that can help alleviate constipation. These include increasing your intake of fiber-rich foods, such as fruits, vegetables, and whole grains, staying hydrated by drinking plenty of water and other fluids, and engaging in regular physical activity to promote healthy digestion.

## Gua Sha for Women's Health

Gua Sha is an ancient Chinese practice that involves scraping the skin with a smooth, flat tool to promote healing, reduce inflammation, and alleviate pain. While the practice is often associated with facial rejuvenation and relaxation, it can also be a useful tool for women's health.

One way that Gua Sha can benefit women is by promoting reproductive health. In Chinese medicine, it is believed that the body's energy, or Qi, flows through specific channels, or meridians, that correspond to different organs and bodily functions. The meridian that corresponds to the uterus and ovaries runs through the lower back and hips, and Gua Sha can help stimulate blood flow and Qi circulation in this area, promoting reproductive health.

Gua Sha can also be used to alleviate menstrual cramps and other symptoms of menstrual discomfort. By stimulating blood flow and relaxing muscles in the lower back and abdomen, Gua Sha can help reduce pain and discomfort associated with menstruation. Some practitioners also believe that Gua Sha can help regulate hormones and improve overall menstrual health.

Pregnant women can also benefit from Gua Sha, as it can help alleviate common pregnancy-related discomforts such as back pain and morning sickness. However, it is important to consult with a healthcare provider before trying Gua Sha during pregnancy, as some techniques and areas of the body may be contraindicated.

Gua Sha can also be a useful tool for menopausal women, as it can help alleviate hot flashes, night sweats, and other symptoms of hormonal imbalance. By promoting blood flow and Qi circulation, Gua Sha can help balance the body's energy and ease symptoms of menopause.

In addition to its reproductive and hormonal benefits, Gua Sha can also be a useful tool for breast health. Breast Gua Sha involves gentle scraping over the breast tissue and lymphatic system, which can help promote lymphatic drainage and improve circulation in the breast tissue. Some practitioners also believe that breast Gua Sha can help reduce the risk of breast cancer by promoting overall breast health.

It is important to note that while Gua Sha can be a useful tool for women's health, it should not be used as a replacement for medical treatment or advice. Women who are pregnant, breastfeeding, or experiencing any unusual symptoms should consult with a healthcare provider before trying Gua Sha or any other alternative therapy.

## Menstrual pain relief

Gua sha, an ancient Chinese therapy, has been used for centuries to alleviate a variety of ailments, including menstrual pain. Menstrual pain, also known as dysmenorrhea, is a common condition experienced by women during their menstrual cycle. It is characterized by cramping and pain in the lower abdomen, lower back, and thighs. While over-the-counter pain medication can be effective in reducing menstrual pain, many women prefer to seek natural alternatives, such as gua sha.

Gua sha is believed to work by increasing blood flow and promoting lymphatic drainage, which helps to reduce inflammation and relieve pain. The therapy involves the use of a gua sha tool, such as a jade or rose quartz stone, to apply pressure to the skin in a stroking motion. This pressure helps to break up stagnation in the body, which is believed to be the underlying cause of many health conditions, including menstrual pain.

One of the primary benefits of gua sha for menstrual pain is its ability to reduce inflammation. Inflammation is a natural response of the body's immune system to injury or infection, but chronic inflammation can lead to a variety of health problems, including menstrual pain. Gua sha helps to reduce inflammation by increasing blood flow to the affected area, which helps to deliver oxygen and nutrients to the tissues and remove waste products. This increased blood flow also helps to promote lymphatic drainage, which can help to reduce swelling and alleviate pain.

In addition to reducing inflammation, gua sha can also help to balance hormones, which can contribute to menstrual pain. Hormonal imbalances, such as those caused by stress, can lead to painful periods. Gua sha helps to balance hormones by reducing stress and promoting relaxation. This is achieved through the pressure and stroking motions of the gua sha tool, which help to release tension and promote a sense of calm.

Gua sha can be used to alleviate menstrual pain in several different ways. One common method is to apply the gua sha tool to the lower abdomen, lower back, and thighs, which are the areas most commonly affected by menstrual pain. The tool is applied in a stroking motion, with gentle pressure, to help increase blood flow and reduce inflammation. This can be done several times a day, as needed, to alleviate pain and discomfort.

Another method of using gua sha for menstrual pain is to combine it with essential oils. Essential oils, such as lavender and clary sage, have been shown to have pain-relieving properties and can be used to enhance the effects of gua sha. A few drops of essential oil can be added to the skin prior to applying the gua sha tool, which helps to enhance the therapeutic effects of the therapy.

It is important to note that gua sha should not be used as a substitute for medical treatment. If menstrual pain is severe or persistent, it is important to consult with a healthcare provider to rule out any underlying medical conditions. However, gua sha can be used as a complementary therapy to help reduce pain and discomfort during the menstrual cycle.

## Supporting pregnancy and postpartum recovery

Gua Sha is an ancient Chinese therapy that has been used for thousands of years to help relieve a variety of ailments. One area where Gua Sha can be particularly effective is in supporting pregnancy and postpartum recovery. Below we will explore how Gua Sha can be used to help women during this transformative time.

During pregnancy, women's bodies go through a lot of changes, both physically and hormonally. These changes can cause discomfort and pain, especially in the back, hips, and legs. Gua Sha can help to alleviate some of these discomforts by improving circulation and reducing inflammation. Additionally, Gua Sha can help to relieve stress and promote relaxation, which can be especially beneficial during pregnancy.

Gua Sha can also be helpful during labor and delivery. The use of Gua Sha on the lower back and hips can help to relieve pain and encourage relaxation during labor. Additionally, Gua Sha can be used to promote cervical ripening and encourage the onset of labor. After delivery, Gua Sha can be used to help with postpartum recovery. Women may experience pain and discomfort in the lower back, hips, and legs, as well as soreness and stiffness in the neck and shoulders from holding and nursing the baby. Gua Sha can be used to alleviate these discomforts and promote healing.

It is important to note that while Gua Sha can be beneficial during pregnancy and postpartum recovery, there are certain precautions that should be taken. Women should only receive Gua Sha from a trained and licensed practitioner who is experienced in working with pregnant and postpartum women. Additionally, certain areas of the body should be avoided during pregnancy, such as the ankles and lower abdomen.

One of the main benefits of Gua Sha for women's health is its ability to support the flow of Qi, or vital energy, throughout the body. In traditional Chinese medicine, it is believed that a blockage or imbalance in the flow of Qi can cause illness and discomfort. Gua Sha works by using a smooth tool, such as a jade or rose quartz gua sha tool, to apply pressure and scrape the skin in a specific pattern. This helps to release tension and promote the flow of Qi and blood in the body.

Gua Sha can be used to help with a variety of conditions that may affect women during pregnancy and postpartum recovery. Some of these conditions include:

1. Back pain: Gua Sha can be used to help relieve pain and stiffness in the back. The tool is applied in a sweeping motion along the spine and surrounding muscles to promote circulation and relieve tension.

2. Swollen feet and ankles: Gua Sha can be used to help reduce swelling in the feet and ankles. The tool is applied in a gentle, sweeping motion along the affected areas to promote circulation and reduce inflammation.

3. Breast engorgement: Gua Sha can be used to help relieve breast engorgement, a common condition that occurs when the breasts become overfull with milk. The tool is applied in a gentle, circular motion over the breast to promote circulation and encourage the flow of milk.

4. Postpartum depression: Gua Sha can be used to help alleviate symptoms of postpartum depression. The tool is applied in a gentle, soothing motion to promote relaxation and reduce stress.

In addition to these conditions, Gua Sha can also be used to help with other issues that may arise during pregnancy and postpartum recovery, such as headaches, constipation, and insomnia.

## Gua Sha for Athletes and Sports Performance

Gua sha is a therapeutic technique that has been used for centuries in traditional Chinese medicine to relieve muscle tension, improve circulation, and promote healing. In recent years, it has gained popularity among athletes and sports enthusiasts for its potential to improve performance and speed up recovery from injuries.

Athletes and sportspeople push their bodies to the limit, subjecting them to intense physical stress and strain. This stress can lead to muscle soreness, stiffness, and inflammation, which can affect performance and increase the risk of injury. Gua sha can be used to address these issues by promoting circulation, reducing muscle tension, and improving flexibility.

One of the key benefits of gua sha for athletes is its ability to increase blood flow to the muscles. When muscles are worked hard during exercise, they can become tight and constricted, which restricts blood flow and oxygen supply. This can lead to muscle soreness and fatigue. By using gua sha to release tension in the muscles, blood flow is increased, allowing more oxygen and nutrients to reach the tissues. This can help to reduce soreness, promote healing, and speed up recovery time.

Gua sha can also be used to improve flexibility and range of motion. Athletes who are more flexible are less prone to injuries because they are able to move their joints through a greater range of motion. By using gua sha to release tension in the muscles and fascia, athletes can improve their flexibility and reduce their risk of injury.

Another benefit of gua sha for athletes is its ability to reduce muscle soreness and inflammation. When muscles are subjected to intense exercise, they can become inflamed, leading to soreness and stiffness. Gua sha can help to reduce inflammation by increasing circulation and promoting the flow of lymphatic fluid. This can help to reduce muscle soreness and promote faster recovery.

Gua sha can also be used to address specific sports-related injuries. For example, it can be used to relieve pain and stiffness in the neck and shoulders caused by repetitive strain injuries from activities such as swimming or cycling. It can also be used to address tennis elbow, plantar fasciitis, and other common sports injuries.

To use gua sha for sports performance, it is important to work with a trained practitioner who understands the specific needs of athletes. They can customize the treatment to address the specific needs of the individual, focusing on areas of tension and soreness.

In addition to its physical benefits, gua sha can also have a positive impact on an athlete's mental well-being. The deep relaxation and stress reduction that can result from a gua sha session can help athletes to feel more focused, calm, and centered, which can improve their performance on the field or in the gym.

## Enhancing performance

Gua sha is a traditional Chinese practice that has been used for centuries to help improve health and well-being. It involves the use of a tool to scrape the skin, which can help to stimulate circulation, relieve tension, and promote relaxation. For athletes, this technique can also provide additional benefits for enhancing performance and improving recovery.

One of the primary benefits of gua sha for athletes is its ability to help alleviate muscle soreness and stiffness. By increasing circulation to the affected area, gua sha can help to flush out toxins and reduce inflammation, which can speed up the recovery process and reduce the risk of injury.

Gua sha can also help to improve flexibility and range of motion, which can be especially beneficial for athletes who need to perform a wide range of movements. By breaking up scar tissue and adhesions in the muscles, gua sha can help to increase mobility and reduce the risk of strains or sprains.

In addition to physical benefits, gua sha can also help athletes to manage stress and improve mental focus. By promoting relaxation and reducing tension, gua sha can help athletes to stay calm and focused during high-pressure situations. This can be particularly helpful for athletes who need to perform at their best under stressful conditions, such as during competition.

There are several different techniques that can be used in gua sha for athletes. One popular approach is to focus on specific areas of the body that are particularly prone to soreness or tension, such as the shoulders, neck, or legs. By targeting these areas with specific strokes and techniques, athletes can help to alleviate pain and improve mobility.

Another effective approach is to incorporate gua sha into a broader recovery routine, such as after a workout or competition. By using gua sha in combination with other techniques such as stretching or massage, athletes can help to further enhance their recovery and reduce the risk of injury.

It is important to note that while gua sha can be highly beneficial for athletes, it is important to use it safely and appropriately. It is recommended to consult with a trained practitioner or coach who can help to ensure that the technique is being used correctly and that it is being used in conjunction with other appropriate recovery techniques.

## Recovery and injury prevention

Gua Sha is a traditional Chinese medicine technique that is gaining popularity in the West for its many benefits, including aiding in injury recovery and injury prevention for athletes. The technique involves using a tool to scrape the skin in a specific pattern to stimulate blood flow and promote healing.

One of the main benefits of Gua Sha for athletes is that it can help with recovery after strenuous activity. When muscles are worked hard during exercise, they can become sore and stiff, making it difficult to continue training. Gua Sha can help to alleviate this soreness by increasing blood flow to the muscles, which can help to flush out waste products like lactic acid that can contribute to soreness.

Another benefit of Gua Sha for athletes is that it can help to prevent injuries. By using the technique regularly, athletes can keep their muscles loose and flexible, which can reduce the risk of strains and sprains. Additionally, Gua Sha can help to break up scar tissue and adhesions in the muscles, which can also reduce the risk of injury.

Gua Sha can be particularly beneficial for athletes who engage in high-impact sports like running or jumping. These types of activities can cause a lot of stress on the joints, which can lead to injuries over time. By using Gua Sha to increase blood flow and reduce inflammation in the joints, athletes can help to prevent these types of injuries from occurring.

In addition to its physical benefits, Gua Sha can also help athletes to improve their mental focus and reduce stress. By stimulating the nervous system and promoting relaxation, Gua Sha can help athletes to feel more calm and centered, which can be particularly beneficial for those who compete in high-pressure environments.

It's important to note that while Gua Sha can be an effective tool for injury recovery and prevention, it should always be used in conjunction with other forms of therapy and under the guidance of a trained professional. Athletes should also be aware of the potential risks associated with Gua Sha, including the possibility of skin irritation or bruising.

## Gua Sha for Chronic Pain and Conditions

Gua Sha, a traditional Chinese medicine technique, is becoming increasingly popular for its benefits in managing chronic pain and conditions. This non-invasive therapy involves using a smooth-edged tool to scrape the skin to stimulate circulation and promote healing. While Gua Sha has been used for centuries, recent research has supported its effectiveness in managing various chronic conditions.

One of the primary benefits of Gua Sha is its ability to reduce inflammation. Chronic inflammation is a common underlying factor in many chronic pain conditions, including arthritis and fibromyalgia. Gua Sha helps to increase circulation and lymphatic drainage, which can reduce inflammation in the affected area. Studies have shown that Gua Sha can significantly reduce pain and stiffness in those with chronic conditions, and the benefits can last for weeks or even months after the treatment.

Gua Sha is also effective in managing chronic neck and back pain. Poor posture, long hours sitting in front of a computer, and other lifestyle factors can lead to chronic pain in the neck and back. Gua Sha can help to alleviate pain and tension in these areas by promoting circulation and reducing muscle stiffness. This can also improve range of motion and flexibility, making it an effective therapy for those with chronic pain and limited mobility.

Fibromyalgia is a chronic pain condition that affects millions of people worldwide. The condition is characterized by widespread pain, fatigue, and cognitive issues. Gua Sha has been shown to be effective in managing fibromyalgia symptoms, including pain and stiffness. In a study of 100 participants with fibromyalgia, those who received Gua Sha therapy reported significant improvements in pain, stiffness, and quality of life compared to those who did not receive the treatment.

Another condition that can be managed with Gua Sha is carpal tunnel syndrome. This condition occurs when the median nerve in the wrist is compressed, causing pain, numbness, and tingling in the hand and wrist. Gua Sha can help to reduce inflammation and improve circulation in the affected area, which can alleviate symptoms and improve overall hand function.

Gua Sha has also been shown to be effective in managing chronic headaches and migraines. The therapy can reduce tension and stiffness in the neck and shoulders, which are common triggers for headaches.

Additionally, Gua Sha can stimulate circulation and promote relaxation, which can also reduce the frequency and intensity of headaches.

Lastly, Gua Sha has been used to manage chronic digestive issues, such as irritable bowel syndrome (IBS) and chronic constipation. Gua Sha can help to improve digestion by stimulating circulation and reducing inflammation in the digestive tract. This therapy can also alleviate symptoms such as abdominal pain, bloating, and constipation.

While Gua Sha has many benefits for managing chronic pain and conditions, it is important to note that it should not be used as a substitute for medical treatment. It is always recommended to speak with a healthcare professional before beginning any new therapy, especially if you have a chronic condition or are taking medication.

## Fibromyalgia

Fibromyalgia is a chronic pain condition that affects millions of people around the world. It is a disorder that causes widespread pain, fatigue, and tenderness in the muscles, joints, and soft tissues. While the exact cause of fibromyalgia is unknown, researchers have suggested that it may be related to abnormal levels of neurotransmitters in the brain, genetic factors, or environmental triggers.

While there is no cure for fibromyalgia, there are many treatments available that can help manage the symptoms. One such treatment is Gua Sha, a traditional Chinese medicine technique that involves scraping the skin with a smooth-edged tool to improve circulation and release tension in the muscles and tissues.

Gua Sha has been shown to be an effective treatment for fibromyalgia, helping to reduce pain and stiffness in the muscles and joints. It works by increasing blood flow to the affected areas, which in turn helps to reduce inflammation and promote healing.

During a Gua Sha session, the practitioner will use a smooth-edged tool, such as a spoon or a jade stone, to gently scrape the skin along the muscles and tissues. This action helps to break up adhesions in the fascia, which are the connective tissues that surround the muscles and organs.

The scraping action of the tool also helps to stimulate the body's natural healing response, triggering the release of endorphins, which are the body's natural painkillers. This helps to reduce pain and improve overall wellbeing.

One of the benefits of Gua Sha is that it is a non-invasive, drug-free treatment option, which is particularly important for those with fibromyalgia who may be sensitive to medications or have concerns about the potential side effects.

Another benefit of Gua Sha is that it is a highly customizable treatment, meaning that the practitioner can tailor the technique to the specific needs of the individual. This may involve using different tools, applying different amounts of pressure, or focusing on specific areas of the body.

In addition to reducing pain and stiffness, Gua Sha has also been shown to be effective in reducing fatigue and improving sleep, both of which are common symptoms of fibromyalgia. By promoting relaxation and reducing stress, Gua Sha can help to improve overall quality of life for those with fibromyalgia.

It is important to note that while Gua Sha can be an effective treatment for fibromyalgia, it should be used in conjunction with other therapies, such as exercise, physical therapy, and medication, as part of a comprehensive treatment plan.

In addition, it is important to work with a qualified practitioner who has experience in treating fibromyalgia with Gua Sha. This will help to ensure that the treatment is safe and effective, and that it is tailored to the individual needs of the patient.

## Arthritis

Arthritis is a chronic condition characterized by inflammation and stiffness in the joints. It can cause severe pain and can limit a person's ability to carry out day-to-day activities. Gua Sha is an ancient Chinese therapy that has been used for centuries to help alleviate pain and inflammation. In recent years, it has gained popularity as a natural treatment option for arthritis.

Gua Sha involves using a tool to scrape the skin in a specific area, usually the affected joint, in order to stimulate blood flow and promote healing. The tool is typically made of materials like jade, rose quartz, or stainless steel, and can come in a variety of shapes and sizes depending on the area being treated.

One of the main benefits of Gua Sha for arthritis is its ability to reduce inflammation. Inflammation is a key factor in arthritis, as it can cause damage to the joints and lead to pain and stiffness. By promoting blood flow and lymphatic drainage, Gua Sha can help to reduce inflammation and alleviate pain.

Another benefit of Gua Sha for arthritis is its ability to improve range of motion in the affected joint. Arthritis can cause stiffness and limited movement in the joints, making it difficult to perform everyday tasks. Gua Sha can help to break up scar tissue and adhesions in the joint, allowing for increased mobility and flexibility.

In addition to its physical benefits, Gua Sha can also have a positive impact on mental health. Chronic pain conditions like arthritis can be mentally exhausting and can lead to anxiety and depression. Gua Sha is a calming and relaxing therapy that can help to reduce stress and promote a sense of well-being.

When using Gua Sha for arthritis, it is important to work with a trained practitioner who can tailor the treatment to your specific needs. They can help to determine the best tools and techniques to use based on the severity and location of your arthritis.

It is also important to note that while Gua Sha can be an effective treatment option for arthritis, it should not be used as a substitute for medical care. Arthritis is a chronic condition that requires ongoing management and treatment, and Gua Sha should be used in conjunction with other therapies as recommended by a healthcare professional.

## Gua Sha for Emotional Well-being

Gua Sha is an ancient Chinese healing technique that has been used for centuries to improve physical health and emotional well-being. While Gua Sha is known for its benefits in addressing physical conditions, such as pain and inflammation, it can also have a positive impact on emotional health. Below we will explore how Gua Sha can help improve emotional well-being, including reducing stress and anxiety, promoting relaxation, and improving sleep.

One of the primary ways that Gua Sha can help improve emotional well-being is by reducing stress and anxiety. Stress is a common experience in modern life, and it can have negative impacts on both physical and mental health. Research has shown that Gua Sha can help reduce stress by lowering levels of the stress hormone cortisol in the body. When cortisol levels are high, we can feel anxious, irritable, and on edge. By reducing cortisol levels, Gua Sha can help us feel more calm and relaxed.

Another way that Gua Sha can help improve emotional well-being is by promoting relaxation. Gua Sha involves using a smooth tool to scrape the skin in a particular pattern, which can help to release tension and tightness in the muscles. This can have a relaxing effect on the body and mind, helping us feel more at ease and peaceful. Additionally, Gua Sha can help promote the flow of energy and blood in the body, which can help to balance the nervous system and reduce feelings of tension and stress.

In addition to reducing stress and promoting relaxation, Gua Sha can also improve sleep. Sleep is essential for overall health and well-being, and poor sleep can have a negative impact on our emotional health. Research has shown that Gua Sha can help improve sleep by reducing pain and promoting relaxation. When we are in pain or feeling tense, it can be difficult to fall asleep and stay asleep. By reducing pain and tension, Gua Sha can help us sleep more soundly and wake up feeling refreshed and rejuvenated.

Another way that Gua Sha can improve emotional well-being is by promoting self-care and self-love. Taking time to care for ourselves is essential for our mental and emotional health, and Gua Sha can be a way to connect with ourselves and show ourselves love and kindness. By taking the time to perform Gua Sha on ourselves, we can slow down and be present in the moment, which can help us feel more connected to ourselves and our emotions.

Finally, Gua Sha can also help improve emotional well-being by promoting a sense of empowerment and control. Chronic pain and illness can leave us feeling helpless and out of control, but by using Gua Sha as a tool for self-care, we can take control of our health and well-being. When we feel in control, we are better able to manage our emotions and navigate the challenges of life.

## Releasing emotional tension

Gua sha is a traditional Chinese medicine technique that involves using a scraping tool to apply pressure and friction to the skin. While it is often used for physical health benefits, such as pain relief and improved circulation, it can also have significant emotional benefits. Below we will explore how Gua sha can be used to release emotional tension.

Emotions can have a significant impact on our physical health. Chronic stress, for example, can lead to a range of health issues, including headaches, muscle tension, and digestive problems. Gua sha can help to alleviate these physical symptoms by promoting relaxation and reducing tension in the body.

One way that Gua sha can release emotional tension is by stimulating the release of endorphins. Endorphins are natural painkillers that are produced by the body in response to certain stimuli, such as exercise, laughter, and massage. When Gua sha is applied to the skin, it stimulates the production of endorphins, which can help to reduce pain and promote a sense of well-being.

Gua sha can also help to release emotional tension by stimulating the parasympathetic nervous system. The parasympathetic nervous system is responsible for the body's rest and digest response, which helps to reduce stress and promote relaxation. When Gua sha is applied to the skin, it stimulates the parasympathetic nervous system, which can help to reduce stress and promote relaxation.

In addition to promoting relaxation and reducing stress, Gua sha can also help to release emotional tension by stimulating the lymphatic system. The lymphatic system is responsible for removing waste and toxins from the body, and when it becomes congested, it can lead to a range of health issues, including fatigue, headaches, and muscle tension. Gua sha can help to stimulate the lymphatic system, which can help to reduce these symptoms and promote a sense of well-being.

Gua sha can also be used to address specific emotional issues. For example, it can be used to help release anger and frustration. When we experience these emotions, we often hold tension in our muscles, which can lead to headaches, neck pain, and other physical symptoms. By applying Gua sha to the affected areas, we can help to release this tension and promote a sense of calm.

Similarly, Gua sha can be used to help release grief and sadness. When we experience these emotions, we often feel a sense of heaviness or tightness in our chest. By applying Gua sha to the chest and upper back, we can help to release this tension and promote a sense of emotional release.

Gua sha can also be used to promote a sense of grounding and connection. When we feel disconnected from ourselves or from others, we often experience physical symptoms, such as anxiety, tension, and fatigue. By applying Gua sha to the feet and lower legs, we can help to promote a sense of grounding and connection, which can help to reduce these symptoms and promote a sense of well-being.

## Balancing emotions

Gua Sha, an ancient Chinese healing technique, is a popular modality used to balance emotions and alleviate physical ailments. This therapy involves scraping the skin with a smooth-edged tool to increase circulation, release toxins, and reduce tension. Below we will discuss how Gua Sha works to balance emotions, and how it can be used to address a range of emotional issues.

According to Chinese medicine, emotions are believed to be closely tied to organ systems in the body. When emotions are not expressed or processed effectively, they can become stuck, leading to physical and emotional imbalances. Gua Sha works by stimulating the flow of Qi, or life force energy, through the body's meridian channels. When the energy is flowing freely, the body can release stuck emotions and restore balance.

One way that Gua Sha can balance emotions is by reducing stress and anxiety. When the body is under stress, the sympathetic nervous system is activated, leading to a range of physical responses such as increased heart rate and shallow breathing. Gua Sha can help to activate the parasympathetic nervous system, which counteracts the stress response and induces relaxation. This can help to reduce anxiety and promote a sense of calm.

Gua Sha can also be effective in releasing anger and frustration. In Chinese medicine, the liver is associated with the emotion of anger, and when the liver is imbalanced, feelings of anger and frustration can arise. Gua Sha applied to the liver meridian can help to release stagnant energy and reduce anger and frustration.

Another emotional issue that Gua Sha can address is depression. Depression is often associated with a lack of energy and motivation, and Gua Sha can help to increase energy levels by improving circulation and stimulating the flow of Qi. Gua Sha can also help to release toxins from the body, which can improve overall physical health and contribute to a sense of well-being.

Gua Sha can also be used to address grief and sadness. The lungs are associated with the emotion of grief, and when the lungs are imbalanced, feelings of sadness can arise. Gua Sha applied to the lung meridian can help to release stagnant energy and promote emotional healing.

In addition to addressing specific emotional issues, Gua Sha can also promote overall emotional well-being. By balancing the body's energy, Gua Sha can help to promote a sense of inner peace and harmony. Gua Sha can also improve sleep quality, which is essential for emotional and mental health.

## Gua Sha for Children and Elderly

Gua Sha is a healing technique that has been used for centuries in traditional Chinese medicine. It involves using a scraping tool to gently massage the skin, which can have a variety of health benefits. While Gua Sha is often associated with adults, it can also be used on children and the elderly. Below we will explore the benefits of Gua Sha for these two groups.

Gua Sha for Children

Gua Sha can be a safe and effective therapy for children, especially those suffering from respiratory illnesses, digestive problems, and skin conditions. The technique involves using a scraping tool to apply pressure to the skin, which can help to stimulate the immune system and promote blood flow. This can be particularly beneficial for children who have weak immune systems or who are prone to illness.

One of the most common uses of Gua Sha for children is for respiratory illnesses such as asthma, bronchitis, and pneumonia. The technique can help to open up the airways and improve lung function, making it easier for children to breathe. Gua Sha can also be used to help alleviate coughing and congestion, which can be especially helpful for young children who may have difficulty sleeping due to these symptoms.

Gua Sha can also be beneficial for children with digestive problems, such as constipation or diarrhea. By stimulating the digestive system, Gua Sha can help to regulate bowel movements and improve overall digestion. In addition, Gua Sha can be used to help relieve stomach pain and discomfort.

Another benefit of Gua Sha for children is its ability to improve skin conditions such as eczema, hives, and rashes. By stimulating blood flow and promoting the removal of toxins from the body, Gua Sha can help to reduce inflammation and improve the appearance of the skin. This can be particularly helpful for children who suffer from skin conditions that can be itchy or painful.

When performing Gua Sha on children, it is important to use a light touch and to be gentle. The technique should never be painful or uncomfortable for the child, and care should be taken to avoid sensitive areas of the body. It is also important to work with a qualified practitioner who has experience working with children.

Gua Sha for the Elderly

Gua Sha can also be a beneficial therapy for the elderly, especially those who suffer from chronic pain, arthritis, and other age-related conditions. As we age, our bodies can become more prone to inflammation and pain, which can be alleviated through the use of Gua Sha.

One of the most common uses of Gua Sha for the elderly is for the treatment of arthritis. Gua Sha can help to reduce inflammation in the joints and improve range of motion, making it easier for seniors to move and perform daily activities. In addition, Gua Sha can help to alleviate pain associated with arthritis, which can be a common issue for seniors.

Gua Sha can also be used to help alleviate chronic pain, such as back pain, neck pain, and headaches. By promoting blood flow and reducing inflammation, Gua Sha can help to reduce pain and discomfort in these areas. This can be especially helpful for seniors who may have limited mobility and who may suffer from pain due to prolonged periods of sitting or standing.

Another benefit of Gua Sha for the elderly is its ability to promote relaxation and reduce stress. By stimulating the nervous system and promoting the release of endorphins, Gua Sha can help to reduce feelings of anxiety and promote a sense of calm. This can be particularly helpful for seniors who may be dealing with the stress of chronic illness or who may be experiencing feelings of isolation or loneliness.

When performing Gua Sha on the elderly, it is important to be gentle and to use a light touch. Seniors may have delicate skin or may be more sensitive to pressure, so care should be

## Gentle techniques

Gua Sha is an ancient healing technique that involves scraping the skin with a tool to promote healing and relaxation. While Gua Sha is often associated with deep tissue massage and trigger point therapy, it can also be used as a gentle technique for children and the elderly. Below we will explore how Gua Sha can benefit these populations and the unique considerations that must be taken into account when using this technique.

Gua Sha has been used for thousands of years to treat a wide range of conditions, from pain and inflammation to respiratory and digestive issues. The technique involves using a smooth-edged tool, such as a jade stone or spoon, to scrape the skin in long strokes. This action stimulates blood flow and releases tension in the muscles, fascia, and connective tissue, which can help to reduce pain and promote relaxation.

For children and the elderly, Gua Sha can be a gentle and effective way to address a variety of health concerns. In children, Gua Sha can be used to alleviate common complaints such as colds, flu, and digestive issues. The technique is gentle and non-invasive, making it well-suited for children who may be hesitant to undergo more traditional forms of treatment.

When performing Gua Sha on children, it is important to use a light touch and to pay close attention to their comfort level. It is also important to use a smaller tool and to avoid applying too much pressure or scraping too deeply. Additionally, it may be helpful to involve the child in the process, explaining what the technique entails and allowing them to choose their preferred tool or essential oil for the treatment.

For the elderly, Gua Sha can be used to address a variety of age-related conditions such as arthritis, muscle stiffness, and respiratory issues. The gentle scraping action of Gua Sha can help to promote circulation and release tension, reducing pain and discomfort in the affected areas.

When performing Gua Sha on the elderly, it is important to take into account any pre-existing medical conditions or medications they may be taking. For example, those taking blood thinners may be at an increased risk of bruising or bleeding, so it may be necessary to use a lighter touch or avoid certain areas of the body. It is also important to make sure that the elderly person is comfortable throughout the treatment and to adjust the pressure and technique as needed.

In addition to its physical benefits, Gua Sha can also be used to support emotional well-being in both children and the elderly. The technique has been shown to promote relaxation and reduce stress and anxiety, which can be particularly beneficial for these populations.

When using Gua Sha for emotional well-being, it may be helpful to incorporate essential oils or aromatherapy into the treatment. Lavender, for example, is known for its calming and relaxing properties, while peppermint can be invigorating and uplifting. It is also important to create a safe and comfortable environment, using soft lighting, soothing music, and comfortable bedding or pillows.

## Benefits for specific age groups

Gua Sha is a traditional Chinese therapy that has been used for thousands of years to treat a variety of health conditions. While it is often associated with muscular and skeletal problems, Gua Sha can also provide a wide range of benefits for people of all ages. Below we will explore the benefits of Gua Sha for specific age groups and how it can help improve their overall health and well-being.

Children:

Gua Sha is a gentle therapy that can be used on children to help improve their immune system, digestion, and respiratory health. It is especially beneficial for children who suffer from frequent colds, allergies, and asthma. Gua Sha can also help children who experience digestive problems such as constipation, diarrhea, or stomach pain. By promoting blood flow and lymphatic drainage, Gua Sha can help alleviate inflammation and promote healing.

Elderly:

As we age, our body's natural healing processes slow down, and we become more prone to a range of health issues. Gua Sha can be an effective therapy for the elderly as it can help alleviate pain, stiffness, and other symptoms associated with conditions such as arthritis, osteoporosis, and chronic pain. It can also help improve mobility and flexibility, promote better sleep, and reduce stress and anxiety. Gua Sha is a safe and gentle therapy that can be used by the elderly to improve their overall health and well-being.

Adults:

Adults can benefit from Gua Sha in a variety of ways, from improving circulation and promoting lymphatic drainage to relieving tension and reducing stress. It can be used to alleviate headaches, migraines, and other chronic pain conditions, as well as to promote healing from injuries and surgeries. Gua Sha can also help improve skin health by promoting blood flow and stimulating collagen production. It can be used to reduce fine lines and wrinkles, improve skin texture, and promote a more youthful appearance.

Pregnant women:

Pregnancy can be a challenging time for women, both physically and emotionally. Gua Sha can be a safe and effective therapy for pregnant women to help alleviate some of the discomforts associated with pregnancy, such as back pain, nausea, and fatigue. It can also help promote better sleep, reduce stress and anxiety, and prepare the body for childbirth. Gua Sha is a gentle therapy that can be used throughout pregnancy to help support the health and well-being of both mother and baby.

Athletes:

Athletes can benefit from Gua Sha to help improve their performance, prevent injuries, and speed up recovery time. It can be used to alleviate muscle soreness, promote better blood flow, and improve flexibility and range of motion. Gua Sha can also help reduce inflammation and promote healing from injuries, such as sprains and strains. By promoting better circulation and lymphatic drainage, Gua Sha can help flush out toxins and waste products, which can help improve overall athletic performance.

## Combining Gua Sha with Other Modalities

Gua sha is an ancient Chinese healing technique that has been used for thousands of years to alleviate various health problems. The technique involves using a smooth-edged tool to scrape the skin, which helps to release tension, improve circulation, and promote healing. Gua sha is often used in conjunction with other modalities, such as acupuncture, massage, and cupping, to enhance their effectiveness.

When combined with acupuncture, gua sha can help to improve the flow of qi, or life force energy, through the body. Acupuncture involves the insertion of fine needles into specific points on the body to stimulate the flow of qi and promote healing. Gua sha can be used to enhance the effects of acupuncture by promoting the movement of blood and lymphatic fluid, which helps to reduce inflammation and pain.

Massage is another modality that can be combined with gua sha to enhance its effectiveness. Massage involves applying pressure to the muscles and soft tissues of the body to promote relaxation and relieve tension. Gua sha can be used to help release tight muscles and knots, allowing the massage therapist to work more effectively.

Cupping is another modality that is often used in conjunction with gua sha. Cupping involves using cups to create suction on the skin, which helps to stimulate blood flow and promote healing. Gua sha can be used before cupping to help warm up the muscles and soft tissues, allowing the cups to be placed more effectively.

In addition to these modalities, gua sha can also be combined with other techniques such as aromatherapy and herbal medicine. Aromatherapy involves using essential oils to promote relaxation and relieve stress. Gua sha can be used to help the essential oils penetrate more deeply into the skin, enhancing their effectiveness.

Herbal medicine is another modality that can be combined with gua sha. Chinese herbal medicine uses a variety of herbs and other natural substances to promote healing and balance in the body. Gua sha can be used to help the herbs penetrate more deeply into the skin, enhancing their effectiveness.

It is important to note that gua sha should only be performed by a trained professional, as improper use of the technique can cause bruising and other injuries. Before undergoing any treatment involving gua sha or other modalities, it is important to consult with a healthcare provider to ensure that it is safe and appropriate for your individual needs.

## Acupuncture

Acupuncture is a traditional Chinese medicine practice that involves inserting thin needles into specific points in the body to stimulate the body's natural healing processes. This modality has been used for thousands of years to treat a variety of conditions and has gained popularity worldwide in recent years. While acupuncture is often used on its own, it can also be combined with other modalities, such as Gua Sha, to enhance its effects.

Gua Sha, another ancient Chinese healing technique, involves using a smooth tool, such as a spoon or stone, to scrape the skin on specific parts of the body. This action is believed to help release stagnation and tension in the muscles and tissues, improving circulation and promoting healing. When combined with acupuncture, Gua Sha can amplify the benefits of the treatment.

One of the primary benefits of combining acupuncture and Gua Sha is increased circulation. Acupuncture needles stimulate the body's blood flow, and Gua Sha helps move the blood and lymphatic fluids throughout the body. This can be especially beneficial for individuals with chronic pain, as poor circulation can lead to stiffness, soreness, and decreased range of motion. By increasing blood flow, acupuncture and Gua Sha can help alleviate these symptoms and promote overall healing.

Another benefit of combining these modalities is the potential to address both acute and chronic conditions. Acupuncture is commonly used to treat acute conditions, such as muscle strains or joint sprains, as well as chronic conditions like arthritis or fibromyalgia. Gua Sha can also be used to address both acute and chronic pain, making it an ideal complement to acupuncture. By working together, these techniques can help provide more comprehensive pain relief for individuals dealing with both short-term and long-term pain.

In addition to physical benefits, combining acupuncture and Gua Sha can also have positive emotional effects. Both modalities work to balance the body's energy, or qi, and promote a sense of relaxation and calmness. This can be especially beneficial for individuals dealing with stress or anxiety, as these conditions can impact both physical and emotional well-being. By promoting relaxation and stress reduction, acupuncture and Gua Sha can help individuals feel more balanced and centered.

While acupuncture and Gua Sha are both safe and effective on their own, combining them can enhance their benefits and provide more comprehensive healing. It's important to work with a qualified practitioner who is trained in both modalities and can create a treatment plan tailored to your specific needs. With the right combination of acupuncture and Gua Sha, you can experience improved circulation, pain relief, and emotional well-being.

## Massage

Massage is a popular form of manual therapy that has been used for centuries to promote relaxation, relieve tension, and improve overall well-being. It involves the manipulation of soft tissues, including muscles, tendons, and ligaments, to help improve circulation, decrease pain, and enhance range of motion. Gua Sha, on the other hand, is a traditional Chinese technique that involves scraping the skin with a smooth-edged tool to improve circulation and relieve tension. When combined, these two modalities can enhance the benefits of each other and provide a more comprehensive approach to healing.

Massage therapy has been used for centuries as a way to promote healing and relaxation. This manual therapy involves the manipulation of soft tissues to improve circulation, decrease pain, and increase range of motion. There are many different types of massage, including Swedish massage, deep tissue massage, and sports massage. Each type of massage involves specific techniques that target different areas of the body and provide different benefits.

Gua Sha, also known as scraping therapy, is a traditional Chinese technique that involves the use of a smooth-edged tool, such as a ceramic spoon, to scrape the skin. This technique is used to promote circulation, relieve tension, and reduce pain. Gua Sha is typically performed on the back, neck, and shoulders, but can be used on other areas of the body as well.

When combined with massage therapy, Gua Sha can enhance the benefits of each modality. The scraping action of Gua Sha can help to release tension and break up adhesions in the muscles and connective tissues, while the massage can help to soothe sore muscles and promote relaxation. By combining these two modalities, patients can experience a more comprehensive approach to healing that addresses both the physical and emotional aspects of pain and tension.

Massage therapy and Gua Sha can also be used in combination with other therapies, such as acupuncture. Acupuncture is a traditional Chinese therapy that involves the insertion of fine needles into specific points on the body to promote healing and balance. When used in combination with massage and Gua Sha, acupuncture can enhance the benefits of each modality and provide a more comprehensive approach to healing.

In addition to massage therapy and acupuncture, Gua Sha can also be used in combination with other complementary therapies, such as herbal medicine and meditation. Herbal medicine involves the use of natural remedies, such as herbs, roots, and flowers, to promote healing and balance in the body. Meditation is a form of mindfulness practice that involves focusing on the present moment to promote relaxation and reduce stress.

## Gua Sha in Professional Practice

Gua Sha, a traditional Chinese therapy, has been gaining popularity in recent years due to its various benefits. In professional practice, Gua Sha is used by licensed professionals such as acupuncturists, massage therapists, and chiropractors. It is often incorporated into treatment plans for a variety of health conditions, including chronic pain, headaches, and digestive issues. Gua Sha is a safe and effective treatment that can help improve overall well-being.

Licensed acupuncturists use Gua Sha to complement acupuncture treatments. It involves the use of a Gua Sha tool to scrape the skin, which is believed to stimulate the flow of blood and energy (qi) in the body. The therapist applies pressure on specific points on the skin, which can help alleviate pain and reduce inflammation. Gua Sha is often used to treat conditions such as neck and back pain, migraines, and digestive issues. It is considered to be a non-invasive and gentle treatment that can produce immediate results.

Massage therapists also incorporate Gua Sha into their practice to help improve circulation and reduce tension in the body. The therapist applies oil to the skin and uses a Gua Sha tool to massage the muscles, helping to release knots and tension. This technique can be especially effective in treating conditions such as plantar fasciitis, carpal tunnel syndrome, and frozen shoulder. Massage therapists may also incorporate Gua Sha into full-body massages to help clients achieve a deeper state of relaxation.

Chiropractors also use Gua Sha as part of their treatment plans. It can be used to help alleviate pain and stiffness in the muscles and joints, and to improve range of motion. Gua Sha can also help to release tension in the fascia, which is a connective tissue that surrounds muscles, bones, and organs. By releasing tension in the fascia, chiropractors can help improve posture and reduce the risk of injury. Gua Sha is often used as a complementary treatment to spinal adjustments and other chiropractic techniques.

In professional practice, Gua Sha is typically used as part of a larger treatment plan that may include other modalities such as acupuncture, massage, and chiropractic adjustments. It is important to consult with a licensed professional before undergoing any type of treatment, including Gua Sha. While Gua Sha is generally considered safe, it may not be suitable for everyone. Individuals with certain medical conditions, such as bleeding disorders or skin infections, should avoid Gua Sha.

## Integrating Gua Sha into your practice

Integrating Gua Sha into your practice can be a valuable addition for any healthcare practitioner looking to expand their skillset and offer their patients a variety of options for wellness and healing. This ancient Chinese therapy has been used for centuries to promote circulation, relieve tension, and alleviate pain. As interest in holistic health and natural remedies grows, more people are turning to Gua Sha as a complementary or alternative treatment.

Gua Sha involves using a smooth-edged tool, such as a ceramic spoon or a jade stone, to apply pressure to the skin and scrape it in a specific pattern. This pressure and scraping can stimulate the immune system, promote lymphatic drainage, and increase blood flow to the affected area, which can help reduce inflammation and pain. Practitioners who use Gua Sha in their practice may find that it can be effective in treating a variety of conditions, including musculoskeletal pain, headaches, digestive issues, and more.

One of the benefits of incorporating Gua Sha into your practice is that it is a non-invasive, low-risk treatment that can be performed on patients of all ages. Additionally, Gua Sha can be easily integrated into other modalities, such as acupuncture or massage, to enhance their therapeutic effects. This can provide patients with a comprehensive treatment plan that addresses their unique needs and concerns.

Before incorporating Gua Sha into your practice, it is important to receive proper training and education in the technique. This will help ensure that you are using the correct tools and techniques, as well as avoiding potential complications. There are several educational resources available, including online courses, workshops, and certification programs. These programs can teach you the proper techniques for using Gua Sha and provide you with the knowledge necessary to safely integrate it into your practice.

Once you have received proper training, you can begin integrating Gua Sha into your practice. It is important to assess each patient's individual needs and determine whether Gua Sha is an appropriate treatment option for them. It is also important to communicate the benefits and potential risks of Gua Sha with your patients and obtain their informed consent before beginning treatment.

During a Gua Sha session, the practitioner will use a smooth-edged tool to apply pressure and scrape the skin in a specific pattern. This pressure and scraping can cause a temporary redness or bruising of the skin, which is a normal response to the treatment. However, it is important to avoid applying too much pressure or scraping too aggressively, as this can cause injury or discomfort to the patient.

After a Gua Sha session, patients may experience some soreness or discomfort in the treated area, which can be relieved with gentle stretching or massage. It is important to advise patients to avoid exposing the treated area to extreme temperatures, such as hot baths or cold compresses, as this can cause further irritation.

## Ethical considerations

Gua sha is an ancient healing technique that has been gaining popularity in recent years as a natural way to alleviate pain and tension in the body. While the technique itself is generally considered safe, there are certain ethical considerations that practitioners and patients should be aware of.

First and foremost, it is important to ensure that gua sha is being performed by a qualified and trained practitioner. While it may seem simple to perform, improper technique or use of tools can result in injury or harm to the patient. Practitioners should be properly licensed or certified in the technique and should have a thorough understanding of human anatomy and any contraindications for gua sha, such as bleeding disorders or certain medications.

Another ethical consideration is informed consent. Patients should be fully informed of the potential benefits and risks of gua sha, as well as any alternatives, before consenting to the treatment. They should also be made aware of any potential discomfort or pain that may occur during the treatment, as well as any potential side effects such as bruising or temporary redness of the skin.

Privacy and modesty are also important considerations. Practitioners should ensure that patients are appropriately draped and comfortable during the treatment, and that any areas of the body not being worked on are covered. Patients should feel safe and respected throughout the treatment process.

It is also important to consider cultural appropriation when using gua sha in a Western context. Gua sha has its roots in traditional Chinese medicine and is deeply rooted in Chinese culture. When using gua sha in a Western context, it is important to acknowledge and respect this cultural heritage and to avoid appropriating or exploiting the practice.

Finally, practitioners should be aware of any potential conflicts of interest. They should avoid making false or exaggerated claims about the benefits of gua sha or using the technique as a way to sell other products or services. The focus should always be on the patient's well-being and providing safe and effective treatment.

## Establishing a Consistent Gua Sha Practice

Establishing a Consistent Gua Sha Practice

Gua Sha is an ancient healing technique that has been used in Traditional Chinese Medicine for centuries. This therapy involves using a smooth-edged tool to apply pressure to the skin, which can help to stimulate blood flow and relieve tension in the muscles. Gua Sha has been shown to be effective in treating a wide range of conditions, from chronic pain and headaches to digestive issues and stress. If you are interested in incorporating Gua Sha into your daily routine, there are several tips that can help you establish a consistent practice.

1. Educate Yourself: The first step in establishing a consistent Gua Sha practice is to educate yourself about the technique. There are many resources available, from books and online tutorials to classes and workshops. It's important to understand the basic principles behind Gua Sha, including the types of tools used, the various techniques involved, and the potential benefits and risks.

2. Invest in Quality Tools: Once you have a basic understanding of Gua Sha, it's time to invest in quality tools. There are many different types of tools available, from traditional jade or rose quartz stones to modern stainless steel devices. It's important to choose a tool that is comfortable to hold and easy to maneuver. Additionally, the tool should be made from high-quality materials to ensure that it lasts for years to come.

3. Develop a Routine: To establish a consistent Gua Sha practice, it's important to develop a routine that works for you. This may involve incorporating Gua Sha into your morning or evening skincare routine, or setting aside a specific time each day to focus on your practice. It's also helpful to establish a consistent technique, using the same strokes and pressure each time you perform the therapy.

4. Practice Regularly: Like any new habit, it takes time and practice to establish a consistent Gua Sha routine. It's important to commit to prac-

ticing regularly, even if it's just a few minutes each day. Consistency is key when it comes to seeing the benefits of Gua Sha, so try to make it a part of your daily routine.

5. Listen to Your Body: It's important to listen to your body when incorporating Gua Sha into your routine. While Gua Sha can be an effective therapy for many people, it's not appropriate for everyone. If you experience any pain or discomfort during your practice, it's important to stop and reassess your technique or seek the guidance of a qualified practitioner.

6. Seek Professional Guidance: If you are new to Gua Sha or have any underlying health conditions, it's important to seek the guidance of a qualified practitioner. They can help you to develop a safe and effective routine that is tailored to your specific needs.

## Tips for success

Gua Sha is a traditional Chinese healing technique that involves scraping the skin with a massage tool to promote circulation and release tension. While it has been used for centuries, it has gained popularity in recent years as a complementary therapy to Western medicine. Whether you are new to Gua Sha or have been practicing for a while, here are some tips to help you establish a consistent and successful Gua Sha practice.

Start with a clean and moisturized face

Before you begin your Gua Sha practice, it is important to start with a clean and moisturized face. This helps to ensure that the massage tool glides smoothly over the skin without causing any irritation or discomfort. Use a gentle cleanser and a lightweight moisturizer to prepare your skin for the massage.

Choose the right massage tool

There are many different types of massage tools available for Gua Sha, including jade, rose quartz, and stainless steel. Choose a tool that feels comfortable in your hand and is easy to use. Some people prefer a smaller tool for more precise movements, while others prefer a larger tool for broader strokes. Experiment with different types of tools to find the one that works best for you.

Use light pressure

When using a massage tool for Gua Sha, it is important to use light pressure. The goal is to promote circulation and release tension, not to cause pain or discomfort. Use gentle, sweeping motions and avoid pressing too hard on the skin. If you feel any discomfort, adjust the pressure or angle of the tool.

Follow a consistent routine

To see the benefits of Gua Sha, it is important to follow a consistent routine. Incorporate Gua Sha into your daily or weekly skincare regimen to see the best results. Start with a few minutes of Gua Sha and gradually increase the time as you become more comfortable with the technique.

Focus on specific areas

While Gua Sha can be used on any part of the body, it is important to focus on specific areas to see the best results. For example, you may want to focus on the jawline and cheekbones to promote lymphatic drainage and reduce puffiness, or on the neck and shoulders to release tension and alleviate headaches. Choose the areas that are most important to you and focus your Gua Sha practice on those areas.

Use in combination with other skincare products

Gua Sha can be used in combination with other skincare products to enhance their effectiveness. For example, you may want to use a facial oil or serum before or after your Gua Sha practice to provide extra hydration and nourishment to the skin. Experiment with different combinations of products to find the ones that work best for your skin.

Practice self-care

Gua Sha is not just a skincare practice, it is also a form of self-care. Take the time to focus on yourself and your well-being while you practice Gua Sha. Create a relaxing environment, play some calming music, and take deep breaths to promote relaxation and reduce stress.

## Overcoming common challenges

Gua sha is a traditional Chinese healing technique that involves the use of a smooth-edged tool to scrape the skin, typically on the back, neck, shoulders, and limbs. The practice is believed to help release tension and improve circulation, leading to a wide range of health benefits. However, as with any form of therapy, there can be challenges that arise. Below we will discuss some common challenges that people may face when incorporating gua sha into their healthcare regimen, as well as strategies for overcoming these challenges.

One of the most common challenges when starting a gua sha practice is learning how to properly use the tool. Gua sha tools come in various shapes and sizes, and it can be difficult to know which one to use for specific areas of the body. Additionally, the technique itself may take some time to master, as it involves applying the correct amount of pressure and angle to the skin. Fortunately, there are many resources available for those looking to learn more about gua sha. Online tutorials and instructional videos can be helpful in demonstrating proper technique, and some practitioners may offer workshops or classes for those looking to receive hands-on instruction.

Another challenge that people may encounter is discomfort or bruising during or after a gua sha session. The pressure applied during the scraping motion can be intense, and some people may experience temporary redness or bruising in the area. It is important to communicate with your practitioner about any discomfort or pain you may be experiencing, as they may be able to adjust their technique to make the experience more comfortable. Additionally, using a lighter touch or shorter sessions may help to reduce any discomfort or bruising.

For those with existing medical conditions or injuries, gua sha may need to be modified or avoided altogether. Certain conditions, such as hemophilia or skin infections, may make gua sha unsafe or inappropriate. It is important to consult with a healthcare professional before beginning a gua sha practice to ensure that it is safe and effective for your individual needs.

Another challenge that people may face is finding the time and space to practice gua sha regularly. Gua sha is most effective when done consistently over time, but it can be difficult to incorporate into a busy schedule. Finding a quiet and comfortable space where you can focus on your practice can be helpful in establishing a consistent routine. Additionally, setting aside a specific time each day for your gua sha practice can help to make it a regular part of your self-care regimen.

Lastly, some people may be hesitant to try gua sha due to a lack of understanding or cultural differences. Gua sha has been used for centuries in Chinese medicine, but it may be unfamiliar to those from different cultural backgrounds. It is important to approach gua sha with an open mind and to be willing to learn about its history and benefits. Additionally, seeking out a practitioner who is knowledgeable and experienced in gua sha can help to provide a greater understanding of the technique and its cultural significance.

## Advanced Gua Sha Techniques

1. Advanced Gua Sha Techniques: Exploring the Depths of Traditional Chinese Medicine

Gua Sha, also known as "scraping," is a traditional Chinese medicine technique used for thousands of years to address various health issues. The practice involves using a tool to scrape the skin gently, which can stimulate blood flow, release toxins, and alleviate pain and tension in the body. However, there is much more to Gua Sha than just scraping the skin. In recent years, advanced Gua Sha techniques have been developed to help patients address complex health issues and achieve optimal well-being.

Advanced Gua Sha techniques are rooted in the principles of traditional Chinese medicine, which views the body as an interconnected system of organs, meridians, and qi (energy). Practitioners who use advanced Gua Sha techniques take a holistic approach to health, examining not only the symptoms but also the underlying causes of illness. By addressing imbalances in the body and promoting the flow of qi, they aim to help patients achieve lasting health and vitality.

One of the key principles of advanced Gua Sha techniques is the concept of "tongue diagnosis." In traditional Chinese medicine, the tongue is considered a microcosm of the body, and its appearance can reveal much about a patient's overall health. An experienced practitioner can look at the shape, color, and coating of the tongue to assess the condition of the organs and meridians, identify any imbalances or deficiencies, and determine the most appropriate course of treatment.

Another important aspect of advanced Gua Sha techniques is the use of specific tools and techniques for different areas of the body. While the basic scraping technique can be used on various parts of the body, advanced practitioners often use different tools and techniques for specific areas. For example, they may use a smaller tool for the face and neck, a larger tool for the back and hips, and a specialized tool for the feet and hands. By using the right tool for the job, practitioners can apply the appropriate amount of pressure and reach deeper layers of tissue, promoting healing and rejuvenation.

Advanced Gua Sha techniques also incorporate a range of other modalities to enhance their effectiveness. For example, practitioners may use acupuncture, herbal medicine, or cupping alongside Gua Sha to address specific health issues. These modalities work together to address imbalances in the body, promoting the flow of qi and enhancing the body's natural healing processes.

One of the most important benefits of advanced Gua Sha techniques is their ability to address complex health issues that may not respond to other treatments. For example, patients with chronic pain, digestive issues, or hormonal imbalances may benefit from advanced Gua Sha techniques, which can help to rebalance the body and promote lasting health. By taking a holistic approach to health and addressing the underlying causes of illness, practitioners of advanced Gua Sha techniques can help patients achieve optimal health and well-being.

However, it's important to note that advanced Gua Sha techniques should only be performed by experienced practitioners who have received specialized training. While basic scraping techniques can be safely performed at home, advanced techniques require a deep understanding of traditional Chinese medicine principles, as well as specialized tools and techniques.

Attempting to perform advanced Gua Sha techniques without proper training can be dangerous and may cause injury.

## Expanding your skillset

Expanding your skillset in the field of traditional Chinese medicine can provide many benefits for both you and your clients. One way to broaden your knowledge and enhance your treatment options is to learn advanced Gua Sha techniques.

Gua Sha, also known as "scraping," is a traditional Chinese medicine technique that involves using a tool to scrape the skin in a specific pattern or direction. This scraping motion is believed to stimulate blood flow and lymphatic drainage, promote healing, and alleviate pain and tension in the body. Advanced Gua Sha techniques build upon these basic principles and can offer additional therapeutic benefits.

One advanced Gua Sha technique is known as "Fei Fu," or "lung and abdomen scraping." This technique involves using a specially designed tool to gently scrape the skin on the chest and abdomen. It is believed to help clear congestion in the lungs, improve breathing, and promote digestion. It may be particularly helpful for individuals with respiratory issues such as asthma or chronic obstructive pulmonary disease (COPD), as well as those with digestive concerns such as bloating or constipation.

Another advanced Gua Sha technique is "Gu Ren," or "bone scraping." This technique involves using a thicker tool to target deeper layers of tissue, including the bones and joints. It is believed to help alleviate chronic pain and tension, promote joint mobility, and improve circulation to affected areas. It may be particularly helpful for individuals with conditions such as arthritis or fibromyalgia.

In addition to these specific techniques, advanced Gua Sha practitioners may also incorporate other modalities into their treatments, such as acupuncture or cupping. This can create a more comprehensive and personalized approach to healing, and may be particularly helpful for individuals with complex or chronic health conditions.

To expand your skillset in Gua Sha and other traditional Chinese medicine techniques, it is important to seek out reputable training programs and continuing education opportunities. Look for courses that are led by experienced practitioners and provide hands-on training in a variety of techniques. It is also important to ensure that any training you receive is in alignment with your state or country's regulations for practice.

As with any new skill or technique, it is important to practice and integrate advanced Gua Sha techniques into your practice gradually and with care. Start by incorporating one or two new techniques into your existing treatments, and gradually build upon your knowledge and skillset over time.

## Specialized tools and approaches

Gua Sha, a traditional Chinese therapy, has gained popularity in recent years as a safe and effective treatment for various health conditions. The technique involves the use of a scraping tool, typically made of jade, to apply pressure and friction on the skin. While Gua Sha can be performed using the fingers, many practitioners prefer to use specialized tools for greater precision and efficacy.

One popular tool is the Gua Sha board, a flat, smooth tool that is used to scrape the skin. These boards are typically made of materials like jade, rose quartz, or stainless steel. The shape of the board varies, with some being rectangular and others having curved or contoured edges to better fit the curves of the body.

Another specialized tool is the Gua Sha comb, which has teeth-like edges that can be used to scrape and stimulate the skin. This tool is particularly useful for treating conditions like hair loss or scalp tension.

In addition to these specialized tools, some practitioners may also use oils or creams to enhance the effects of Gua Sha. These products can help to lubricate the skin and improve the glide of the tool, making it easier to apply pressure and friction.

While Gua Sha is often used as a standalone therapy, it can also be combined with other modalities for greater effect. For example, Gua Sha may be used in conjunction with acupuncture to improve the flow of energy in the body and enhance the effects of the treatment. Similarly, Gua Sha may be used before or after a massage to help loosen tight muscles and improve circulation.

## Gua Sha for Insomnia and Sleep Disorders

Gua sha, an ancient Chinese healing technique, is becoming increasingly popular in the Western world for its numerous health benefits. One area where gua sha has shown promise is in addressing insomnia and sleep disorders. Insomnia affects millions of people worldwide, and while medication can help, it's not always the best solution. Below we will we'll explore how gua sha can be used to alleviate sleep problems, its benefits, and how to incorporate it into your routine.

Insomnia is a common sleep disorder characterized by difficulty falling or staying asleep, waking up frequently during the night, and waking up too early. While it's a temporary condition for some, others may struggle with it for months or even years. Insomnia can lead to several physical and mental health problems, including fatigue, depression, anxiety, and poor concentration.

Gua sha is an ancient Chinese technique that involves scraping the skin with a smooth tool, such as a ceramic spoon or a jade stone, to stimulate blood flow and lymphatic drainage. When done correctly, gua sha can reduce muscle tension, improve circulation, and promote relaxation, making it an effective treatment for insomnia.

Gua sha is believed to work by stimulating the parasympathetic nervous system, which is responsible for controlling the body's rest and relaxation response. This system helps reduce stress and anxiety, which are common causes of insomnia. By stimulating this system, gua sha can help calm the mind, reduce tension in the body, and promote a sense of relaxation.

Gua sha can also help alleviate physical symptoms that contribute to insomnia, such as muscle tension and pain. The technique works by increasing blood flow to the muscles, which can help reduce inflammation and speed up the healing process. This can lead to reduced muscle tension and pain, allowing for more restful sleep.

There are several gua sha techniques that can be used to address insomnia and sleep disorders. One popular technique is to target specific acupressure points on the body. These points are believed to correspond to different parts of the body and can be used to address specific issues, such as stress, anxiety, or muscle tension.

For example, the acupoint located on the inner wrist, known as the Shen Men or "Spirit Gate," is believed to help calm the mind and promote relaxation. By using gua sha to stimulate this point, you can help reduce stress and anxiety, making it easier to fall asleep.

Another technique involves targeting the neck and shoulders, where tension often accumulates. Gua sha can be used to release tension in these areas, allowing for more restful sleep.

It's important to note that while gua sha can be beneficial for insomnia and sleep disorders, it's not a cure-all solution. Other lifestyle changes, such as improving sleep hygiene, avoiding caffeine and alcohol, and establishing a regular sleep schedule, are also important for addressing insomnia.

Incorporating gua sha into your routine is easy and can be done at home. You'll need a gua sha tool, such as a ceramic spoon or a jade stone, and a lubricant, such as oil or lotion, to glide the tool over the skin. Before beginning, it's essential to warm up the muscles with a warm towel or hot shower to help loosen any tension.

To perform gua sha on the body, apply the lubricant to the targeted area, and use the tool to scrape the skin in a smooth, fluid motion. Apply light to medium pressure, being careful not to cause any pain or discomfort. You can repeat this process several times, gradually increasing the pressure as needed.

For acupressure points, use the gua sha tool to apply pressure to the targeted area, holding for several seconds before releasing. Repeat as needed, applying gentle pressure.

## Techniques for better sleep

Getting a good night's sleep is essential for overall health and well-being. Unfortunately, many people struggle with insomnia and other sleep disorders, which can significantly impact their quality of life. While there are various medications and therapies available to address these issues, some people prefer natural approaches to sleep improvement, such as Gua Sha.

Gua Sha is a traditional Chinese therapy that involves using a smooth tool to scrape the skin in a specific pattern. This practice is believed to improve circulation, relieve pain, and promote overall health and wellness. When it comes to sleep, Gua Sha can be a helpful tool for achieving a restful and restorative night's rest.

One of the ways Gua Sha can improve sleep is by reducing tension in the body. Insomnia and other sleep disorders are often associated with stress and anxiety, which can cause tension to build up in the muscles and soft tissues. Gua Sha can help alleviate this tension by stimulating the body's natural healing response and promoting relaxation.

Another way Gua Sha can improve sleep is by promoting circulation. When we are sleeping, our bodies are repairing and regenerating, and adequate circulation is essential for this process. Gua Sha can improve circulation by increasing blood flow and lymphatic drainage, which helps to remove waste and toxins from the body.

There are several techniques for using Gua Sha to improve sleep. One approach is to focus on the neck and shoulders, as tension in these areas can contribute to insomnia and other sleep disorders. Using a Gua Sha tool, apply gentle pressure in a downward motion along the sides of the neck and across the tops of the shoulders. This can help to release tension and promote relaxation in these areas.

Another technique is to use Gua Sha on the feet. The feet contain numerous pressure points that are connected to different parts of the body, including the organs and glands that regulate sleep. By stimulating these points with Gua Sha, you can promote overall relaxation and help the body prepare for sleep.

It's important to note that Gua Sha is not a substitute for professional medical care, and it's always best to consult with a healthcare provider if you are experiencing chronic sleep issues or other health concerns. However, incorporating Gua Sha into your self-care routine can be a helpful tool for promoting relaxation and restful sleep.

In addition to Gua Sha, there are several other natural approaches to improving sleep. Some people find that practicing relaxation techniques such as meditation, yoga, or deep breathing can be helpful for reducing stress and promoting relaxation. Others find that creating a relaxing bedtime routine, such as taking a warm bath or reading a book, can help signal to the body that it's time to wind down for sleep.

## Establishing a bedtime routine

Establishing a Bedtime Routine for Better Sleep

Getting a good night's sleep is essential for overall health and well-being. Poor sleep quality or insomnia can lead to a host of health problems, including obesity, depression, and cardiovascular disease. Establishing a bedtime routine is a great way to improve your sleep quality and promote better overall health.

The first step in establishing a bedtime routine is to set a regular bedtime and wake-up time. Going to bed and waking up at the same time every day helps to regulate your body's internal clock, making it easier to fall asleep and wake up in the morning.

Next, consider incorporating relaxation techniques into your bedtime routine. Gua sha, a traditional Chinese medicine technique, is one such technique that can help promote relaxation and improve sleep quality.

Gua sha involves the use of a smooth-edged tool, such as a spoon or specialized gua sha tool, to gently scrape the skin in long strokes. The technique is believed to promote blood flow and lymphatic drainage, as well as reduce muscle tension and inflammation.

To incorporate gua sha into your bedtime routine, start by choosing a comfortable and quiet location. Apply a few drops of massage oil or lotion to the area of your body that you want to work on, such as your neck, shoulders, or back. Using a gua sha tool, apply gentle pressure and scrape the skin in long strokes, always moving in the same direction. Be sure to avoid areas of broken skin or inflammation.

In addition to gua sha, there are several other relaxation techniques that you can incorporate into your bedtime routine. Meditation, deep breathing exercises, and yoga are all effective ways to reduce stress and promote relaxation.

It's also important to create a sleep-conducive environment. This means keeping your bedroom dark, quiet, and cool. Invest in a comfortable mattress and pillows, and avoid using electronics in the bedroom.

Establishing a relaxing bedtime routine can help you fall asleep faster and stay asleep longer. It can also help to reduce stress and promote better overall health. Try incorporating gua sha and other relaxation techniques into your bedtime routine and see how it can improve your sleep quality and well-being.

## Gua Sha for Headaches and Migraines

Gua Sha is a traditional Chinese medicine technique that has been used for centuries to treat various conditions, including headaches and migraines. This technique involves the use of a smooth-edged tool, usually made of jade or other materials, to scrape the skin in a specific pattern. The goal of Gua Sha is to improve circulation, release tension and promote healing.

Headaches and migraines can be debilitating and have a significant impact on a person's quality of life. According to the World Health Organization, headaches are one of the most common disorders of the nervous system, affecting up to 50% of the adult population worldwide. Migraines are a type of headache that is typically characterized by severe pain, sensitivity to light and sound, and nausea.

Gua Sha can be an effective treatment for both headaches and migraines. It works by increasing circulation and promoting the flow of Qi, or vital energy, throughout the body. This can help to relieve tension and reduce inflammation, which are two of the main causes of headaches and migraines.

One of the most effective ways to use Gua Sha for headaches and migraines is to focus on the neck and shoulders. Tension in these areas can often contribute to the development of headaches and migraines. By using Gua Sha to release tension and increase circulation in the neck and shoulders, it is possible to reduce the frequency and intensity of headaches and migraines.

To perform Gua Sha on the neck and shoulders, begin by applying a small amount of oil or lotion to the skin. This will help to prevent friction and make it easier to glide the Gua Sha tool across the skin. Next, use the tool to scrape the skin in a downward motion, starting at the base of the neck and moving towards the shoulders. Repeat this motion several times, gradually increasing the pressure as needed.

It is important to be gentle when using Gua Sha, especially in sensitive areas such as the neck and shoulders. If you experience any discomfort or pain, stop immediately and consult with a trained practitioner.

In addition to using Gua Sha on the neck and shoulders, it is also possible to use this technique on the forehead and temples. This can help to relieve tension and reduce inflammation in these areas, which are common triggers for headaches and migraines.

To use Gua Sha on the forehead and temples, begin by applying a small amount of oil or lotion to the skin. Next, use the Gua Sha tool to scrape the skin in a downward motion, starting at the center of the forehead and moving towards the temples. Repeat this motion several times, gradually increasing the pressure as needed.

It is important to note that Gua Sha should not be used as a substitute for medical treatment for headaches and migraines. If you experience frequent or severe headaches or migraines, it is important to consult with a healthcare provider to determine the underlying cause and develop an appropriate treatment plan.

In addition to using Gua Sha, there are several other techniques that can be helpful in managing headaches and migraines. These include practicing relaxation techniques such as meditation and deep breathing, avoiding triggers such as certain foods and stress, and getting regular exercise and adequate sleep.

## Identifying headache triggers

Headaches are a common ailment that can be caused by various factors. Identifying the triggers of a headache can be helpful in preventing future occurrences. Below we will discuss how to identify headache triggers and how Gua Sha can help alleviate headaches.

Firstly, it is important to understand that there are many different types of headaches. Some common types include tension headaches, migraines, and cluster headaches. Each type has its own set of triggers and symptoms. Therefore, it is important to identify the type of headache one is experiencing in order to properly identify the triggers.

One of the most common triggers for headaches is stress. Stress can cause tension in the muscles of the head, neck, and shoulders, leading to tension headaches. Identifying sources of stress and finding ways to manage stress can be helpful in preventing tension headaches.

Another common trigger for headaches is dehydration. When the body is dehydrated, it can lead to headaches. Drinking plenty of water throughout the day can help prevent headaches caused by dehydration.

Certain foods and drinks can also trigger headaches. Common culprits include caffeine, alcohol, and processed foods. Keeping a food diary and noting when headaches occur can help identify which foods may be triggering headaches.

Environmental factors can also contribute to headaches. Bright lights, loud noises, and strong odors can all trigger headaches in some individuals. Identifying and avoiding these triggers can help prevent headaches.

Now that we have discussed some common headache triggers, let's discuss how Gua Sha can be used to alleviate headaches. Gua Sha is a traditional Chinese medicine technique that involves scraping the skin with a smooth tool, such as a jade stone. This technique is believed to help release tension in the muscles and promote circulation.

When it comes to headaches, Gua Sha can be particularly helpful for tension headaches. By applying gentle pressure to the neck, shoulders, and scalp, Gua Sha can help release tension in the muscles that may be contributing to the headache. Additionally, the increased circulation that Gua Sha promotes can help reduce inflammation, which can also contribute to headaches.

It is important to note that Gua Sha should only be performed by a trained practitioner. The technique involves applying pressure to the skin, which can cause bruising if done incorrectly. Therefore, it is important to seek out a qualified practitioner to perform Gua Sha.

In addition to Gua Sha, there are other natural remedies that can be helpful in alleviating headaches. These include:

1. Acupuncture: Similar to Gua Sha, acupuncture is a traditional Chinese medicine technique that involves the insertion of small needles into specific points on the body. Acupuncture is believed to help regulate the flow of energy in the body and promote healing.

2. Massage: Gentle massage can help release tension in the muscles and promote relaxation. This can be particularly helpful for tension headaches.

3. Essential oils: Certain essential oils, such as lavender and peppermint, are believed to have pain-relieving properties. Applying these oils topically or inhaling their scent can help alleviate headaches.

## Effective Gua Sha techniques

Gua Sha is an ancient Chinese technique that involves using a smooth-edged tool to scrape the skin in a specific pattern, in order to stimulate blood flow and promote healing. While this technique has been traditionally used to treat a wide range of ailments, it has gained increasing popularity in recent years as a natural method for alleviating headaches and migraines.

Gua Sha is believed to work by releasing stagnant energy and increasing blood circulation in the affected areas. This can help to relieve tension and pain, as well as promote the body's natural healing processes. When used on the head and neck area, Gua Sha can be particularly effective in treating headaches and migraines.

There are a number of different Gua Sha techniques that can be used to treat headaches and migraines. One of the most common is the "scraping" technique, which involves using a smooth-edged tool to gently scrape the skin in a specific pattern along the affected area. This technique can help to release tension and promote blood flow, which can alleviate headache pain.

Another effective Gua Sha technique for headaches and migraines is the "cupping" technique. This involves using a special cup-shaped tool to create a suction effect on the skin. This can help to stimulate blood flow and reduce tension in the affected area, which can help to alleviate headache pain.

In addition to these techniques, there are a number of other Gua Sha approaches that can be used to treat headaches and migraines. These may include using herbal oils or topical analgesics to enhance the effects of the treatment, or incorporating other traditional Chinese medicine techniques such as acupuncture or acupressure.

One of the key benefits of using Gua Sha to treat headaches and migraines is that it is a non-invasive and natural approach that does not rely on medication or other interventions that may have unwanted side effects. In addition, Gua Sha is a relatively simple and affordable treatment that can be easily incorporated into a daily routine.

To maximize the benefits of Gua Sha for headaches and migraines, it is important to use the technique consistently and in conjunction with other healthy lifestyle practices. This may include incorporating regular exercise, maintaining a healthy diet, and getting enough sleep and rest.

It is also important to identify and address any underlying causes of headaches and migraines, such as stress, poor posture, or other health issues. By combining Gua Sha with other natural and holistic approaches, individuals can achieve a comprehensive and effective treatment plan for managing headaches and migraines.

## Gua Sha for Skin Health

Gua Sha is a traditional Chinese medical technique that involves scraping the skin with a smooth-edged tool to stimulate the flow of blood and qi (life force energy). While it is commonly used for pain relief and relaxation, Gua Sha can also have a positive impact on skin health. Below we will explore the benefits of Gua Sha for the skin, the different techniques used, and how to incorporate it into your daily skincare routine.

One of the primary benefits of Gua Sha for the skin is improved circulation. When the skin is scraped with a Gua Sha tool, it helps to increase blood flow and oxygenation to the area. This increased circulation can help to promote skin cell regeneration and improve skin texture and tone. In addition, Gua Sha can help to reduce inflammation and swelling, which can be especially helpful for those with acne-prone or sensitive skin.

Another benefit of Gua Sha for the skin is lymphatic drainage. The lymphatic system is responsible for removing toxins and waste products from the body, and Gua Sha can help to stimulate lymphatic flow and drainage. This can be especially beneficial for reducing puffiness and dark circles under the eyes, as well as promoting a healthy, glowing complexion.

There are several different techniques used for Gua Sha on the skin. One of the most common is to use a flat, smooth-edged tool to gently scrape the skin in an upward and outward motion. This technique is often used on the face and neck, and can be done with a variety of different tools, including jade, rose quartz, or metal.

Another technique for Gua Sha on the skin involves using a serrated tool to lightly scrape the skin in a back-and-forth motion. This technique is often used on the body to help relieve tension and pain in the muscles and joints.

When incorporating Gua Sha into your daily skincare routine, it is important to start with clean, dry skin. Apply a facial oil or serum to help the tool glide smoothly over the skin, and then use gentle, upward strokes to scrape the skin in the desired areas. It is important to use light pressure and to avoid any areas of the skin that are broken or irritated.

While Gua Sha can be beneficial for the skin, there are also some potential risks to be aware of. If the technique is done too aggressively or with too much pressure, it can cause bruising, redness, or even broken blood vessels. It is important to use caution and to consult with a trained practitioner before attempting Gua Sha on the skin.

## Improving skin texture and elasticity

Gua Sha, an ancient healing technique, has been gaining popularity in recent years as a natural and effective way to improve skin texture and elasticity. This technique involves scraping a smooth tool over the skin in order to promote circulation, reduce inflammation, and stimulate collagen production. Gua Sha has been used for centuries in traditional Chinese medicine to promote overall health and wellness, but its benefits for skin health are becoming increasingly recognized.

One of the main benefits of Gua Sha for skin health is its ability to promote circulation. As the tool is scraped over the skin, it creates micro-trauma that stimulates blood flow to the area. This increased circulation can bring more oxygen and nutrients to the skin cells, helping to nourish and revitalize the complexion. Additionally, this increased blood flow can help to remove toxins and waste products from the skin, which can contribute to a dull, lackluster appearance.

In addition to promoting circulation, Gua Sha can also reduce inflammation in the skin. Inflammation is a major contributor to a wide range of skin concerns, including acne, rosacea, and eczema. By reducing inflammation, Gua Sha can help to calm and soothe the skin, reducing redness and irritation. This can be especially beneficial for those with sensitive skin or inflammatory skin conditions.

Another way that Gua Sha can improve skin health is by stimulating collagen production. Collagen is a protein that is essential for healthy, youthful-looking skin. As we age, our bodies produce less collagen, which can lead to fine lines, wrinkles, and sagging skin. By stimulating collagen production, Gua Sha can help to firm and plump the skin, reducing the appearance of fine lines and wrinkles.

To get the most out of Gua Sha for skin health, it is important to use the proper technique. A smooth, flat tool is typically used, such as a jade or rose quartz gua sha tool. The tool is held at a 45-degree angle and scraped over the skin in an upward and outward motion. It is important to use light pressure and to avoid scraping too hard, as this can cause bruising or other damage to the skin. The technique should be gentle and soothing, rather than aggressive or painful.

In addition to using Gua Sha as a standalone treatment, it can also be combined with other skincare techniques for even greater benefits. For example, Gua Sha can be used after applying a facial oil or serum, which can help to boost absorption and enhance the effects of the product. Gua Sha can also be used in conjunction with facial massage, which can help to further promote circulation and lymphatic drainage.

There are some precautions that should be taken when using Gua Sha for skin health. Those with active acne or other inflammatory skin conditions should avoid using Gua Sha over active breakouts, as this can exacerbate the inflammation. Additionally, those with very thin or delicate skin should use caution, as Gua Sha can be too stimulating for these skin types. It is always a good idea to consult with a skincare professional before trying Gua Sha or any new skincare technique.

## Addressing skin conditions like acne and eczema

Gua Sha is an ancient Chinese therapy that has been used for thousands of years to promote healing, reduce pain, and improve overall well-being. In recent years, it has gained popularity in the West as a complementary therapy for various health conditions, including skin conditions like acne and eczema. Below we will explore the benefits of Gua Sha for skin health, with a focus on how it can help address acne and eczema.

Gua Sha involves using a tool to scrape the skin, typically along the meridian lines of the body. The scraping action helps to increase circulation, release tension and promote lymphatic drainage, which can help to eliminate toxins and reduce inflammation in the body. Gua Sha can be done on the face or body, and it can be used to address a variety of skin concerns.

Acne is a common skin condition that affects millions of people around the world. It is caused by a combination of factors, including excess oil production, clogged pores, inflammation, and bacteria. While there are many over-the-counter treatments available for acne, some people may prefer to try a more natural approach. Gua Sha can be an effective complementary therapy for acne, as it helps to increase circulation and lymphatic drainage, which can help to reduce inflammation and clear toxins from the skin.

When using Gua Sha for acne, it is important to use a light touch and avoid applying too much pressure to the skin. This can cause irritation and make acne worse. Instead, gently scrape the skin in upward motions, working from the center of the face outward. Focus on areas where acne is most prevalent, such as the chin, nose, and forehead.

In addition to promoting circulation and lymphatic drainage, Gua Sha can also help to stimulate collagen production, which can help to improve the texture and elasticity of the skin. This can be particularly beneficial for people with acne scars, as it can help to reduce the appearance of scarring over time.

Eczema is another common skin condition that can be difficult to manage. It is characterized by red, itchy, and inflamed patches of skin, and it can be caused by a variety of factors, including genetics, allergies, and environmental triggers. While there is no cure for eczema, there are a number of treatments available that can help to reduce symptoms and improve quality of life.

Gua Sha can be an effective complementary therapy for eczema, as it helps to reduce inflammation and promote lymphatic drainage, which can help to alleviate symptoms. When using Gua Sha for eczema, it is important to use a gentle touch and avoid scraping over areas of broken or inflamed skin. Instead, focus on areas that are not affected by eczema, such as the arms and legs.

In addition to using Gua Sha, there are a number of other natural remedies that can help to alleviate eczema symptoms. These include using moisturizers to keep the skin hydrated, avoiding harsh soaps and detergents, and identifying and avoiding triggers like stress, certain foods, and environmental allergens.

## Gua Sha for Weight Management

Gua Sha is a traditional Chinese healing practice that involves scraping the skin with a smooth-edged tool to promote healing and wellness. While most commonly used for pain relief and stress reduction, Gua Sha can also be used to support weight management.

The body's lymphatic system plays a critical role in weight management, as it helps to remove waste and toxins from the body. When the lymphatic system is not functioning properly, it can result in fluid retention, bloating, and other symptoms that make weight management more difficult.

Gua Sha has been shown to help stimulate the lymphatic system, allowing it to function more efficiently. By using a Gua Sha tool to massage specific areas of the body, such as the abdomen and legs, it is possible to help promote lymphatic flow and reduce inflammation in these areas.

In addition to promoting lymphatic flow, Gua Sha can also help to improve digestion, another key component of weight management. By using Gua Sha to massage the stomach and intestinal area, it is possible to help improve digestion, reduce bloating and gas, and improve overall gut health.

Furthermore, Gua Sha can help to reduce stress, a common cause of weight gain. When the body is under stress, it produces the hormone cortisol, which can contribute to weight gain and make it more difficult to lose weight. Gua Sha has been shown to help reduce cortisol levels, promoting relaxation and reducing stress.

One study published in the Journal of Traditional Chinese Medicine found that Gua Sha was effective in reducing body mass index (BMI), waist circumference, and body fat percentage in overweight and obese adults. Participants in the study received Gua Sha treatments twice a week for five weeks, along with dietary and exercise counseling. At the end of the study, significant improvements in weight and body composition were observed.

While Gua Sha can be an effective tool for weight management, it is important to remember that it is not a quick fix or a substitute for healthy lifestyle habits. In order to see lasting results, it is important to maintain a healthy diet, exercise regularly, and prioritize stress reduction.

When incorporating Gua Sha into a weight management routine, it is important to work with a qualified practitioner who can provide guidance and support. Gua Sha should not be used on broken skin, and certain areas of the body, such as the face and neck, require specialized techniques and tools.

In addition to in-person treatments, there are also Gua Sha tools that can be used at home for self-massage. These tools are typically made of materials like jade or rose quartz and can be used to massage specific areas of the body to promote lymphatic flow and reduce inflammation.

## Enhancing metabolism

Gua Sha, a traditional Chinese medicine technique, has been used for centuries to treat various health issues, including weight management. Gua Sha involves scraping the skin with a smooth-edged instrument to promote blood circulation, release tension, and stimulate the body's natural healing processes. By applying Gua Sha to specific areas of the body, practitioners believe they can enhance metabolism, leading to improved weight management. Below we will explore the science behind how Gua Sha enhances metabolism and its potential benefits for weight management.

Metabolism refers to the chemical processes in the body that convert food into energy. An individual's metabolism rate is determined by various factors, including age, sex, body composition, and genetics. A faster metabolism rate means that the body burns more calories, which can aid in weight management. Therefore, enhancing metabolism is crucial for weight loss or maintenance.

Gua Sha works by stimulating the circulatory system, which includes the blood vessels, lymphatic vessels, and lymph nodes. Gua Sha creates an increased blood flow to the skin, which can cause capillaries to dilate and increase blood flow to the targeted area. This increase in blood flow can help to remove toxins and other waste products from the body, leading to improved metabolism.

Moreover, Gua Sha can also help to reduce stress, which is known to affect metabolism negatively. Stress releases hormones like cortisol, which can increase the body's production of glucose, leading to weight gain. Gua Sha can help reduce stress by releasing tension in the muscles and promoting relaxation, which can help improve metabolism.

Gua Sha can also aid in digestion and nutrient absorption. Poor digestion can slow down the metabolism, leading to weight gain. By applying Gua Sha to the abdominal area, it can stimulate the digestive system and increase the production of digestive enzymes, leading to improved digestion and nutrient absorption.

There are various Gua Sha techniques that can aid in weight management. One of the most effective techniques is to apply Gua Sha to the abdominal area. The abdominal area is home to several vital organs, including the stomach, liver, and intestines, which play a crucial role in digestion and metabolism. By applying Gua Sha to the abdominal area, it can stimulate these organs and improve digestion, leading to improved metabolism.

Another technique is to apply Gua Sha to the arms and legs, targeting specific acupuncture points. Acupuncture points are specific points on the body that are believed to correspond to different organs and functions in the body. By stimulating these points, it can help to regulate the functions of these organs, leading to improved metabolism and weight management.

It is worth noting that Gua Sha should not be used as a standalone method for weight management. It is important to combine Gua Sha with a healthy diet and regular exercise to achieve maximum benefits. Gua Sha can aid in weight management, but it is not a substitute for a healthy lifestyle.

## Supporting a healthy weight loss journey

Gua Sha, an ancient Chinese healing technique, has gained popularity in recent years for its many health benefits, including weight management. Gua Sha involves using a tool to scrape the skin in specific areas of the body, stimulating circulation and promoting the body's natural healing processes. While it is not a weight-loss miracle, Gua Sha can support a healthy weight loss journey by enhancing metabolism, reducing stress, and improving overall wellness.

One of the ways Gua Sha can aid in weight management is by enhancing metabolism. The technique increases blood flow to the targeted areas, which can stimulate the lymphatic and digestive systems. This increased circulation can help to speed up the metabolism and assist the body in burning calories more efficiently. Additionally, Gua Sha can help to break down fat cells, making them easier for the body to eliminate. By supporting a healthy metabolism, Gua Sha can help individuals reach their weight loss goals more effectively.

Another way Gua Sha can support weight management is by reducing stress levels. Stress is a common contributor to weight gain, as it can increase cortisol levels, leading to cravings for sugary or fatty foods. Gua Sha has been shown to decrease cortisol levels, promoting relaxation and reducing stress. By reducing stress levels, Gua Sha can help individuals make healthier food choices and better manage their weight.

Gua Sha can also improve overall wellness, which is important for individuals on a weight loss journey. The technique can boost immunity, improve sleep quality, and increase energy levels, all of which can support a healthy lifestyle. By promoting overall wellness, Gua Sha can help individuals feel more motivated and energized to make healthy choices and stick to their weight loss goals.

While Gua Sha can be beneficial for weight management, it is important to note that it is not a standalone solution. A healthy diet and regular exercise are essential for achieving and maintaining a healthy weight. Gua Sha can be used as a complementary therapy to support a healthy weight loss journey, but it should not be relied upon as the sole method of weight loss.

To incorporate Gua Sha into a weight loss routine, individuals can use the technique on areas of the body that tend to hold onto fat, such as the thighs, hips, and abdomen. It is recommended to use Gua Sha for at least 10 minutes a day, several times a week, to see results. It is important to use gentle pressure and avoid scraping too hard, as this can cause bruising or damage to the skin. Additionally, drinking plenty of water before and after the treatment can help to flush out toxins and support overall wellness.

## Gua Sha for Mental Health

Gua Sha, an ancient traditional Chinese medicine technique, has been gaining popularity worldwide due to its therapeutic benefits. While primarily known for its physical benefits, Gua Sha can also have a positive impact on mental health. This technique involves using a smooth-edged tool to scrape the skin's surface, stimulating circulation and reducing inflammation, leading to improved mood and relaxation. Here we will discuss the benefits of Gua Sha for mental health.

One of the primary benefits of Gua Sha for mental health is its ability to reduce stress and anxiety. Research has shown that Gua Sha can lower levels of cortisol, the stress hormone, in the body. When cortisol levels are high, it can lead to increased stress and anxiety, which can have a detrimental effect on mental health. Gua Sha can help to counteract this by reducing cortisol levels, leading to a sense of calm and relaxation.

Gua Sha can also have a positive impact on depression. It is believed that Gua Sha can stimulate the release of endorphins, the body's natural mood-boosting chemicals. Endorphins can help to improve mood, reduce stress, and increase overall feelings of well-being. By stimulating the release of endorphins, Gua Sha can help to alleviate symptoms of depression.

Another benefit of Gua Sha for mental health is its ability to improve sleep quality. Poor sleep quality can have a significant impact on mental health, leading to increased stress and anxiety. Gua Sha can help to promote relaxation, leading to better sleep quality. Additionally, Gua Sha can help to alleviate tension in the body, which can contribute to better sleep quality.

Gua Sha can also help to improve focus and concentration. When the body is under stress, it can be challenging to focus and concentrate, leading to decreased productivity and increased anxiety. Gua Sha can help to reduce stress, leading to increased focus and concentration.

Furthermore, Gua Sha can help to improve overall feelings of well-being. By reducing stress and anxiety and promoting relaxation, Gua Sha can help to improve overall mental health. It can also help to promote a sense of self-care and self-love, leading to increased feelings of happiness and contentment.

When incorporating Gua Sha into a self-care routine, it is essential to remember that it is not a substitute for professional mental health treatment. While Gua Sha can have significant benefits for mental health, it should be used in conjunction with other therapies, such as psychotherapy or medication, when necessary.

## Reducing anxiety and depression

Gua sha is an ancient Chinese healing technique that involves the use of a smooth-edged tool to scrape the skin gently. This method is known for its ability to reduce tension in the body, improve blood circulation, and boost the immune system. In recent years, there has been growing interest in the use of gua sha for mental health, particularly for reducing anxiety and depression.

Anxiety and depression are two of the most common mental health disorders worldwide, affecting millions of people. These conditions can be debilitating and have a significant impact on a person's quality of life. While there are various treatments available, many people are turning to complementary and alternative therapies, such as gua sha, to alleviate their symptoms.

Gua sha is believed to work by releasing tension and promoting the flow of energy, or qi, in the body. This can help to regulate the nervous system and reduce feelings of stress and anxiety. The technique is also thought to stimulate the release of endorphins, the body's natural painkillers, which can produce a sense of relaxation and wellbeing.

There are several gua sha techniques that can be used to target anxiety and depression. One approach involves focusing on the neck and shoulders, where tension tends to accumulate. The therapist will use a gua sha tool to gently scrape the skin in upward strokes, working from the base of the neck up to the hairline. This technique can help to release tension in the muscles and promote relaxation.

Another technique involves targeting specific acupressure points on the body. Acupressure is a traditional Chinese medicine practice that involves applying pressure to specific points on the body to stimulate the flow of energy. By combining gua sha with acupressure, therapists can target specific points that are believed to help alleviate anxiety and depression.

In addition to its potential therapeutic benefits, gua sha can also be a soothing and grounding experience for those struggling with mental health issues. The gentle scraping sensation can help to create a sense of calm and relaxation, which can be especially beneficial for those experiencing heightened levels of stress and anxiety.

It is worth noting that while gua sha can be a helpful complementary therapy for mental health, it should not be used as a substitute for professional medical treatment. Those experiencing severe symptoms should always consult with a mental health professional to receive appropriate care.

Gua sha should also be performed by a trained and licensed therapist. While it is generally a safe and non-invasive technique, improper use of the gua sha tool can cause skin irritation and other side effects. It is important to seek out a qualified practitioner who has experience with gua sha and understands how to use the technique safely and effectively.

## Promoting mental clarity

Gua Sha is a traditional Chinese healing technique that has been used for centuries to promote physical, emotional, and mental well-being. While it is commonly known for its ability to relieve physical pain and tension, Gua Sha can also be effective in promoting mental clarity and reducing anxiety and depression.

Gua Sha works by applying pressure to the skin and muscles with a smooth-edged tool, such as a jade stone or a metal scraper. This pressure helps to release tension and improve circulation, which can have a positive impact on both physical and mental health. In terms of mental health, Gua Sha can be particularly effective in promoting relaxation and reducing stress.

Stress is a major contributor to mental health issues, including anxiety and depression. When we experience stress, our bodies release the hormone cortisol, which can have negative effects on our mental and physical health over time. By promoting relaxation and reducing stress, Gua Sha can help to lower cortisol levels and support overall mental well-being.

In addition to promoting relaxation, Gua Sha can also help to improve mental clarity. When we are feeling anxious or depressed, our thoughts can become muddled and it can be difficult to focus. By promoting better circulation and oxygenation to the brain, Gua Sha can help to clear our minds and improve cognitive function. This can help us to better manage our thoughts and emotions, and make clearer decisions.

While Gua Sha can be effective on its own in promoting mental health, it can also be used in conjunction with other treatments or therapies. For example, it can be used in combination with acupuncture, massage, or aromatherapy to enhance their effectiveness in promoting mental well-being.

If you are interested in trying Gua Sha for mental health, it is important to seek out a qualified practitioner who is trained in the technique. They can help you to develop a treatment plan that is tailored to your specific needs and goals. It is also important to maintain a consistent practice to experience the full benefits of Gua Sha over time.

In terms of self-care, there are also ways to incorporate Gua Sha into your daily routine to support mental well-being. For example, you can use a Gua Sha tool to gently massage your temples or the back of your neck to promote relaxation and reduce tension. You can also use it to massage your face and promote lymphatic drainage, which can help to reduce puffiness and improve skin health. Additionally, incorporating Gua Sha into a bedtime routine can be particularly effective in promoting relaxation and better sleep.

## Gua Sha for Respiratory Health

Gua Sha, a traditional Chinese medicine technique, has been gaining popularity in recent years due to its numerous health benefits. In addition to its benefits for the skin, digestion, and emotional well-being, Gua Sha can also be used to support respiratory health.

Respiratory health is a vital aspect of overall health and well-being. Poor respiratory health can result in difficulty breathing, chronic coughing, and even serious conditions such as asthma and pneumonia. Gua Sha can help to promote respiratory health by relieving tension in the muscles, reducing inflammation, and increasing circulation to the lungs and airways.

Gua Sha can be particularly effective for individuals with asthma or other respiratory conditions. In a study published in the Journal of Asthma, researchers found that Gua Sha therapy was effective in improving lung function and reducing asthma symptoms in adults with asthma. The study participants received Gua Sha therapy once a week for eight weeks, and the results showed significant improvement in lung function and a reduction in asthma symptoms.

Gua Sha can also be helpful for individuals with allergies. Allergies can cause inflammation and irritation in the respiratory system, leading to symptoms such as coughing, sneezing, and difficulty breathing. Gua Sha can help to reduce inflammation and relieve tension in the muscles surrounding the airways, making it easier to breathe.

In addition to its benefits for respiratory health, Gua Sha can also be used to support the immune system. The immune system plays a critical role in fighting off infections and other diseases. When the immune system is weak, individuals may be more susceptible to respiratory infections such as the flu and pneumonia.

Gua Sha can help to boost the immune system by increasing circulation and promoting lymphatic drainage. The lymphatic system is responsible for removing toxins and waste from the body, and a healthy lymphatic system can help to support overall immune function.

There are several Gua Sha techniques that can be used to support respiratory health. One technique involves gently scraping the skin on the back and sides of the neck to help relieve tension in the muscles that support the respiratory system. Another technique involves applying pressure to specific points on the chest and back to help open up the airways and promote circulation to the lungs.

It is important to note that Gua Sha should always be performed by a trained professional. While Gua Sha is generally safe, there is a risk of bruising or other skin irritation if the technique is not performed correctly. Additionally, individuals with certain medical conditions such as blood clotting disorders should avoid Gua Sha or consult with their healthcare provider before undergoing the treatment.

## Alleviating asthma and bronchitis

Gua Sha is an ancient technique that has been used for thousands of years in traditional Chinese medicine. It involves the use of a smooth-edged tool, usually made of jade or rose quartz, to scrape the skin in specific areas of the body. Gua Sha is known for its ability to promote healing and well-being, and it can be used to address a wide range of health issues, including respiratory problems like asthma and bronchitis.

Asthma and bronchitis are both respiratory conditions that can cause a range of symptoms, including wheezing, coughing, and shortness of breath. These conditions can be triggered by a variety of factors, including environmental irritants, allergens, and stress. While conventional treatments for these conditions typically involve the use of medications like bronchodilators and corticosteroids, some people find that complementary therapies like Gua Sha can be helpful in managing their symptoms.

Gua Sha works by promoting circulation and stimulating the immune system, which can help to reduce inflammation and improve lung function. It can also help to relax the muscles of the chest and back, which can make it easier to breathe. Additionally, Gua Sha can help to reduce stress and anxiety, which are both common triggers for respiratory conditions.

To use Gua Sha for respiratory health, the therapist will typically focus on the back and chest areas. The therapist will apply oil or lotion to the skin to help the tool glide smoothly, and then use the tool to scrape the skin in a specific pattern. This pattern is designed to promote circulation and encourage the movement of lymphatic fluid, which can help to flush toxins and other waste products out of the body.

During a Gua Sha session, the therapist will also work on acupressure points that are related to the respiratory system. These points are located along the meridians or energy channels that run through the body, and are believed to be connected to specific organs and bodily functions. By working on these points, the therapist can help to rebalance the flow of energy in the body and promote overall health and well-being.

In addition to Gua Sha, there are a number of other complementary therapies that can be helpful for respiratory conditions. Acupuncture, for example, can be used to stimulate specific points in the body that are related to the respiratory system. Herbal medicine can also be helpful, as many herbs have natural anti-inflammatory and expectorant properties.

It is important to note that while Gua Sha and other complementary therapies can be helpful for managing respiratory conditions, they should not be used as a substitute for conventional medical care. If you are experiencing symptoms of asthma or bronchitis, it is important to seek medical attention from a qualified healthcare provider.

## Strengthening the lungs

Gua sha is an ancient healing technique that has been used for centuries to improve physical and mental health. In recent years, it has gained popularity as a complementary therapy for a variety of health issues. One area where gua sha has shown promise is in supporting respiratory health.

Respiratory health is essential for our well-being, as the lungs play a crucial role in supplying oxygen to the body and removing carbon dioxide. Respiratory illnesses such as asthma, bronchitis, and pneumonia can have a significant impact on our health and quality of life.

Gua sha has been shown to be effective in alleviating respiratory symptoms and improving lung function. The technique involves scraping the skin with a smooth-edged tool, which stimulates blood flow and promotes healing. Gua sha can be used on the back, chest, and neck to help alleviate respiratory symptoms such as coughing, wheezing, and shortness of breath.

One study found that gua sha was effective in reducing asthma symptoms in children. The study, published in the Journal of Complementary and Alternative Medicine, showed that children who received gua sha treatments had a significant reduction in the severity and frequency of asthma symptoms. The researchers suggest that gua sha may help improve lung function and reduce inflammation, both of which can contribute to asthma symptoms.

Gua sha has also been found to be effective in reducing symptoms of chronic bronchitis. A study published in the Journal of Traditional Chinese Medicine found that gua sha was effective in reducing cough and improving lung function in patients with chronic bronchitis. The researchers suggest that gua sha may help improve the circulation of the lungs, which can reduce inflammation and promote healing.

In addition to its benefits for specific respiratory conditions, gua sha can also help strengthen the lungs and improve overall respiratory health. By stimulating blood flow, gua sha can help improve oxygenation of the blood and promote the removal of toxins from the lungs.

To incorporate gua sha into your respiratory health routine, you can start by using a gua sha tool on the chest and back. Gently scrape the skin using long strokes, starting from the center of the chest and moving outwards. You can also use circular motions on the upper back to help loosen any tension or congestion.

It is important to note that gua sha should not be used as a replacement for medical treatment for respiratory conditions. If you have a respiratory condition, it is important to seek medical advice from a healthcare professional before trying any complementary therapies.

## Gua Sha for Detoxification

Gua Sha is a traditional Chinese healing technique that has been used for centuries to improve overall health and wellbeing. In recent years, it has gained popularity as a natural detoxification method. Gua Sha involves scraping the skin with a smooth-edged tool to promote the movement of blood and lymphatic fluid, which can help eliminate toxins from the body. Below we will explore the benefits of Gua Sha for detoxification and how it works.

Toxins are all around us in our environment and food, and they can accumulate in our bodies over time, leading to a range of health issues. Detoxification is the process of removing these toxins from the body, and it is an essential aspect of maintaining optimal health. Gua Sha can be a powerful tool in supporting the body's natural detoxification processes.

One of the primary benefits of Gua Sha for detoxification is that it stimulates the lymphatic system. The lymphatic system is responsible for removing waste and toxins from the body, and when it is not functioning correctly, toxins can build up and lead to illness. Gua Sha helps to stimulate the lymphatic system, promoting the movement of lymphatic fluid and the elimination of toxins.

Gua Sha also helps to increase circulation and oxygenation in the body. When the body has better circulation, it is better able to transport oxygen and nutrients to cells and eliminate waste products. This can help to support the body's natural detoxification processes, as well as improve overall health and wellbeing.

Another benefit of Gua Sha for detoxification is that it can help to improve digestion. When the digestive system is functioning correctly, it is better able to eliminate waste products and toxins from the body. Gua Sha can help to stimulate digestion and improve bowel movements, which can aid in the elimination of toxins.

Gua Sha can also be beneficial for the skin, which is the body's largest organ and an essential aspect of the body's natural detoxification processes. The scraping action of Gua Sha can help to improve blood flow and lymphatic drainage in the skin, promoting the elimination of toxins through the skin.

To get the most benefits from Gua Sha for detoxification, it is essential to use the technique correctly. The first step is to choose a high-quality Gua Sha tool, such as a jade or rose quartz tool, which will provide a smooth and gentle scraping action. It is also important to use a good quality oil, such as coconut or jojoba oil, to lubricate the skin and facilitate the movement of the tool.

To perform Gua Sha for detoxification, begin by applying a small amount of oil to the skin. Then, using light pressure, gently scrape the skin in long, sweeping motions, starting at the center of the body and moving outwards towards the limbs. Focus on areas of the body where toxins may accumulate, such as the back, shoulders, and abdomen.

It is important to be gentle when performing Gua Sha, especially on sensitive areas of the body. It is also essential to listen to the body and adjust the pressure and speed of the scraping as necessary to avoid causing pain or discomfort.

In addition to using Gua Sha for detoxification, there are other things that individuals can do to support their body's natural detoxification processes. Eating a healthy diet rich in fruits and vegetables, drinking plenty of water, getting regular exercise, and avoiding exposure to environmental toxins are all important aspects of maintaining optimal health.

## Supporting liver and kidney function

Gua Sha is a traditional Chinese healing technique that involves the use of a smooth-edged tool to scrape the skin in a specific pattern. It has been used for centuries to promote healing and balance within the body, and in recent years, it has gained popularity in the West as a natural and effective way to support detoxification. Gua Sha can be particularly beneficial for supporting liver and kidney function, which are essential organs for the body's natural detoxification processes.

The liver is responsible for filtering toxins from the blood, while the kidneys filter waste products from the body's fluids. When these organs are not functioning optimally, toxins can build up in the body, leading to a wide range of health problems. Gua Sha can help to support the liver and kidneys by improving circulation and lymphatic drainage, which can help to eliminate toxins from the body more effectively.

One of the key benefits of Gua Sha for detoxification is its ability to improve circulation. The scraping action of the tool stimulates the flow of blood and lymphatic fluid in the body, which can help to remove waste products and toxins from the tissues. This increased circulation can also help to bring more oxygen and nutrients to the cells, supporting overall health and vitality.

In addition to improving circulation, Gua Sha can also help to stimulate the lymphatic system. The lymphatic system is a network of vessels and organs that helps to eliminate waste products and toxins from the body. When the lymphatic system is not functioning properly, toxins can build up in the tissues, leading to inflammation and other health problems. Gua Sha can help to stimulate the lymphatic system, helping to improve the body's natural detoxification processes.

Gua Sha can also be beneficial for supporting the liver and kidneys directly. By scraping along the sides of the spine and other specific acupressure points, Gua Sha can help to promote the flow of energy through these organs, supporting their function and helping to eliminate toxins from the body.

Another benefit of Gua Sha for detoxification is its ability to reduce inflammation in the body. Chronic inflammation is a common problem in many health conditions, and it can interfere with the body's natural detoxification processes. Gua Sha has been shown to help reduce inflammation by increasing circulation and lymphatic drainage, as well as by releasing tension and promoting relaxation in the body.

There are many different approaches to using Gua Sha for detoxification, depending on the specific health concerns and goals of the individual. Some practitioners may recommend using Gua Sha in conjunction with other detoxification techniques, such as dietary changes, herbal remedies, or other therapies. Others may focus on specific acupressure points or patterns to target the liver and kidneys directly.

To get the most benefit from Gua Sha for detoxification, it is important to work with a trained practitioner who can provide guidance on the most effective techniques and approaches for your individual needs. It is also important to stay well-hydrated and to support the body's natural detoxification processes with a healthy diet and lifestyle.

## Eliminating toxins from the body

Gua Sha is an ancient healing technique that has been used for thousands of years to promote health and wellness. One of the most significant benefits of Gua Sha is its ability to help eliminate toxins from the body. Toxins can build up in the body from a variety of sources, including pollution, processed foods, and even stress. If left unchecked, these toxins can lead to a range of health problems, including chronic diseases. Fortunately, Gua Sha can help the body eliminate these toxins and restore balance to the body.

The liver and kidneys are the two primary organs responsible for eliminating toxins from the body. The liver filters toxins from the blood, while the kidneys filter toxins from the urine. When these organs are overworked or not functioning correctly, toxins can build up in the body, leading to a range of health problems. Gua Sha can help support the liver and kidneys' function, allowing them to work more efficiently and effectively.

One way that Gua Sha can help eliminate toxins from the body is by increasing circulation. The technique involves using a tool, such as a smooth-edged stone or metal instrument, to scrape the skin in a specific pattern. This scraping action stimulates the skin and underlying tissues, increasing blood flow and lymphatic drainage. Improved circulation and lymphatic drainage can help remove toxins from the body more efficiently, reducing the burden on the liver and kidneys.

Gua Sha can also help promote sweating, another way the body eliminates toxins. Sweating helps to flush toxins out of the body through the skin. Gua Sha can promote sweating by stimulating the skin and underlying tissues, increasing circulation, and raising body temperature. This increased sweating can help eliminate toxins from the body and support overall health.

Another way Gua Sha can help eliminate toxins from the body is by promoting relaxation and reducing stress. Stress can negatively impact the body's ability to eliminate toxins by suppressing the immune system and decreasing circulation. Gua Sha can help promote relaxation by stimulating the nervous system and reducing muscle tension. This relaxation response can help reduce stress and support the body's natural detoxification processes.

Finally, Gua Sha can help improve digestion, another critical factor in eliminating toxins from the body. When the digestive system is not functioning correctly, toxins can build up in the body, leading to a range of health problems. Gua Sha can help improve digestion by stimulating the digestive organs and increasing circulation to the gut. This increased circulation can help promote healthy digestion and elimination, reducing the burden on the liver and kidneys.

## Gua Sha for Eye Health

Gua Sha is an ancient Chinese technique used to promote healing and wellness. While it is commonly associated with muscle and joint pain relief, it can also be used to improve eye health. Gua Sha involves the use of a smooth tool, such as a jade or rose quartz stone, to gently massage the skin and underlying tissues. The technique is believed to improve circulation and lymphatic drainage, which can help to reduce inflammation and promote healing.

One of the key benefits of Gua Sha for eye health is improved circulation. Poor circulation can lead to a range of eye problems, including dry eyes, blurry vision, and even glaucoma. By increasing circulation to the eyes, Gua Sha can help to reduce inflammation and promote healing. Additionally, Gua Sha can help to stimulate the lymphatic system, which can help to remove toxins and waste products from the body.

Another benefit of Gua Sha for eye health is stress relief. Stress is a common cause of eye strain and can lead to a range of eye problems, including headaches, blurred vision, and dry eyes. Gua Sha can help to reduce stress and tension in the body, which can help to alleviate these symptoms.

Gua Sha can also be used to treat specific eye conditions, such as macular degeneration and cataracts. Macular degeneration is a common age-related eye condition that affects the retina and can lead to vision loss. Gua Sha can help to improve circulation to the retina, which can help to slow down the progression of the disease. Similarly, Gua Sha can be used to treat cataracts, which are caused by a buildup of protein in the lens of the eye.

By promoting circulation and lymphatic drainage, Gua Sha can help to remove these protein deposits and improve overall eye health.

To perform Gua Sha for eye health, a smooth tool, such as a jade or rose quartz stone, is gently massaged around the eye area. The tool should be used in a gentle, circular motion, starting from the inner corner of the eye and moving outward. It is important to avoid applying too much pressure or pulling on the skin, as this can cause irritation and damage.

It is also important to note that Gua Sha should not be used as a substitute for professional medical care. If you are experiencing any eye problems or have a pre-existing eye condition, it is important to consult with a qualified healthcare professional before attempting Gua Sha or any other self-care technique.

In addition to Gua Sha, there are a number of other self-care techniques that can be used to improve eye health. These include:

1. Eye exercises: Regular eye exercises can help to improve circulation to the eyes and reduce strain and tension.

2. Proper nutrition: A healthy diet rich in vitamins and minerals, particularly vitamin A and omega-3 fatty acids, can help to support eye health.

3. Rest and relaxation: Getting enough rest and taking breaks from activities that require intense visual focus, such as reading or using a computer, can help to reduce eye strain and promote healing.

## Relieving eye strain and dryness

Gua Sha is an ancient healing technique that involves using a smooth-edged tool to scrape the skin, primarily on the back, neck, and shoulders. However, it is not limited to these areas and can also be used on other parts of the body, including the face and around the eyes. Gua Sha for eye health has become increasingly popular in recent years due to its potential benefits for relieving eye strain and dryness.

Eye strain and dryness are common problems in today's world, as many people spend a significant amount of time looking at screens, whether it be for work or leisure activities. Eye strain can cause discomfort, headaches, and blurred vision, while dryness can lead to irritation, redness, and even infections. Gua Sha can be a natural and effective way to help alleviate these symptoms.

Gua Sha works by stimulating circulation and promoting lymphatic drainage, which can help to reduce inflammation and improve blood flow to the affected area. This increased circulation can help to nourish the eyes and promote healing.

To perform Gua Sha for eye health, a small Gua Sha tool can be used to gently scrape the skin around the eyes. This should be done with light pressure and in a slow and controlled manner to avoid any discomfort or damage to the delicate skin in this area. It is important to avoid any contact with the eyeball itself.

A common technique used in Gua Sha for eye health is to start at the inner corner of the eye and work outward, following the curve of the eyebrow. The tool should be held at a slight angle and moved in a gentle scraping motion, repeating this process several times. The same technique can be used under the eye, starting at the inner corner and moving outward.

Another technique that can be used in Gua Sha for eye health is to massage the temples. The temples are located at the side of the head, just above the ears, and are often a point of tension for many people. Massaging the temples can help to reduce stress and tension in the head and promote relaxation.

While Gua Sha can be a beneficial practice for promoting eye health, it is important to remember that it is not a substitute for professional medical treatment. If you are experiencing severe or persistent symptoms related to eye strain or dryness, it is important to seek medical advice.

In addition to Gua Sha, there are other things you can do to support eye health. These include taking regular breaks from screen time, using proper lighting, and staying hydrated. A healthy diet that includes plenty of fruits and vegetables can also help to support eye health, as can getting enough sleep and exercise.

## Improving vision and eye-related issues

Gua Sha is an ancient Chinese practice that involves using a tool to scrape the skin to promote healing and wellness. While it is often associated with pain relief and relaxation, it also has potential benefits for eye health. Below we will explore the ways in which Gua Sha can help relieve eye strain and dryness, as well as improve vision and address eye-related issues.

Eye strain and dryness are common issues in our digital age. Staring at a computer or smartphone screen for extended periods can cause fatigue, discomfort, and dryness of the eyes. Gua Sha can be used to alleviate these symptoms by stimulating blood flow and promoting relaxation. By using a Gua Sha tool along the eyebrows, cheekbones, and temples, practitioners can help increase circulation to the eyes, which can help reduce inflammation and dryness. Additionally, Gua Sha can promote relaxation of the surrounding muscles, reducing tension that can contribute to eye strain and discomfort.

In addition to relieving eye strain and dryness, Gua Sha can also help improve vision. This is because the practice can help stimulate the flow of energy, or Qi, throughout the body. According to traditional Chinese medicine, the eyes are connected to the liver, and a healthy liver is essential for good vision. By using Gua Sha on specific acupressure points on the face, practitioners can help improve liver function and promote healthy vision. Additionally, Gua Sha can help reduce inflammation in the eyes, which can contribute to conditions like macular degeneration and cataracts.

Gua Sha can also be used to address specific eye-related issues. For example, it can be effective in treating puffy eyes, dark circles, and crow's feet. Puffiness and dark circles are often caused by poor circulation and fluid retention in the face, while crow's feet are a result of the skin losing elasticity over time. By using Gua Sha to stimulate circulation and promote lymphatic drainage in the face, practitioners can help reduce puffiness and dark circles, as well as tighten and firm the skin, reducing the appearance of wrinkles and fine lines.

It is worth noting that while Gua Sha can be effective in promoting eye health, it should not be used as a replacement for traditional medical care. If you have a serious eye condition or are experiencing significant vision problems, it is important to consult a medical professional before attempting any self-treatment.

When incorporating Gua Sha into your routine for eye health, it is important to use the proper technique and tools. There are specific Gua Sha tools designed for use on the face, and practitioners should use gentle pressure and avoid applying too much force. It is also important to avoid using Gua Sha on any broken or irritated skin, as well as areas that have undergone recent surgery or cosmetic treatments.

## Gua Sha for Hormonal Balance

Gua Sha is an ancient Chinese practice that involves scraping the skin to stimulate circulation and promote healing. While it's often associated with pain relief, Gua Sha has also been shown to have a positive effect on hormonal balance. Below we will explore how Gua Sha can help to regulate hormones and promote overall health and well-being.

Hormonal imbalances can affect people of all ages and genders, and can lead to a wide range of symptoms and health issues. Common hormonal imbalances include thyroid disorders, adrenal fatigue, PCOS, and menopause. These conditions can cause symptoms such as fatigue, weight gain, mood swings, insomnia, and more.

Gua Sha works by stimulating the body's natural healing response and improving circulation. When the skin is scraped, it causes micro-traumas that trigger an inflammatory response. This inflammation stimulates blood flow, which helps to deliver oxygen and nutrients to the affected area. The increased blood flow also helps to remove metabolic waste and toxins from the body.

One way that Gua Sha can help to balance hormones is by improving thyroid function. The thyroid gland produces hormones that regulate metabolism and energy levels. When the thyroid gland is not functioning properly, it can cause a range of symptoms, including fatigue, weight gain, and mood swings. Research has shown that Gua Sha can help to stimulate the thyroid gland and improve thyroid function, which can lead to improved energy levels and overall health.

Gua Sha can also be beneficial for women experiencing hormonal imbalances related to menopause or menstrual cycles. Menopause is a natural part of the aging process, but can cause a range of symptoms including hot flashes, mood swings, and insomnia. Gua Sha can help to stimulate blood flow to the ovaries, which can help to regulate hormones and reduce menopausal symptoms. Similarly, women who experience painful or irregular periods may benefit from Gua Sha, as it can help to improve blood flow to the reproductive organs and balance hormone levels.

In addition to its hormonal balancing effects, Gua Sha has also been shown to have a positive effect on the immune system. When the body is under stress, the immune system can become compromised, leading to a range of health issues. Gua Sha helps to reduce stress and improve circulation, which can boost the immune system and improve overall health.

There are a variety of Gua Sha techniques that can be used to promote hormonal balance. One common technique is to scrape along the spine and neck, as this area is rich in nerve endings and can help to stimulate the thyroid gland. Another technique is to scrape the abdomen, which can help to improve digestion and stimulate the reproductive organs. Other techniques may target specific acupressure points or meridians, depending on the individual's specific hormonal imbalances.

It's important to note that Gua Sha should always be performed by a trained professional, as improper technique can lead to bruising or other injuries. Additionally, while Gua Sha can be a helpful tool for balancing hormones and improving overall health, it should not be used as a replacement for medical treatment. Anyone experiencing symptoms of a hormonal imbalance should consult with their healthcare provider to determine the best course of treatment.

## Regulating hormones

Gua Sha is a traditional Chinese therapy that involves scraping the skin with a smooth-edged tool to promote circulation, relieve pain, and improve overall health. While most people associate Gua Sha with physical benefits, such as muscle tension relief, it can also be a valuable tool for promoting hormonal balance.

Hormonal imbalances can occur due to various factors such as stress, diet, and lifestyle changes, and can lead to a range of symptoms, including irregular periods, mood swings, weight gain, and acne. Fortunately, Gua Sha can help regulate hormones and promote overall hormonal health.

One of the primary ways Gua Sha works to regulate hormones is by reducing stress. Stress is a significant contributor to hormonal imbalances, and Gua Sha is known to reduce stress levels by promoting relaxation and improving mood. During a Gua Sha session, the therapist will use the tool to apply pressure to specific areas of the body, such as the neck, shoulders, and upper back, to release tension and promote relaxation. This, in turn, can help regulate hormones such as cortisol and adrenaline, which are associated with the body's stress response.

Gua Sha can also be effective in promoting hormonal balance by increasing circulation. The therapy stimulates blood flow to the targeted areas, which can help regulate hormones such as estrogen and progesterone, responsible for regulating menstrual cycles in women. This can be especially beneficial for women experiencing irregular periods or premenstrual syndrome (PMS) symptoms, such as bloating, cramping, and mood swings.

Another way Gua Sha can help regulate hormones is by promoting detoxification. Hormonal imbalances can result from toxins in the body that interfere with the endocrine system, which produces and regulates hormones. Gua Sha can help eliminate toxins by promoting lymphatic drainage, which involves stimulating the lymphatic system to remove waste and excess fluids from the body. This, in turn, can help regulate hormones such as estrogen and testosterone, which are processed by the liver and eliminated through the lymphatic system.

In addition to its physical benefits, Gua Sha can also promote emotional well-being, which can have a significant impact on hormonal health. Gua Sha promotes relaxation and reduces stress, which can lead to improved mood and overall emotional balance. This, in turn, can positively impact hormonal health by reducing cortisol levels, promoting better sleep, and improving overall quality of life.

To incorporate Gua Sha into a hormone-balancing routine, it's important to work with a qualified practitioner who can provide personalized recommendations based on individual needs and concerns. Gua Sha can be used on various parts of the body, including the face, neck, and back, and can be combined with other holistic therapies, such as acupuncture and herbal remedies, for a comprehensive approach to hormonal health.

## Supporting adrenal health

Gua Sha is an ancient Chinese healing practice that has been used for thousands of years to address a variety of health concerns. Among its many benefits, Gua Sha has been found to support adrenal health and help regulate hormones. Below we will explore how Gua Sha can support adrenal health, as well as the mechanisms behind its ability to regulate hormones.

The adrenal glands are two small glands located above the kidneys that are responsible for producing hormones such as cortisol, adrenaline, and aldosterone. These hormones play a critical role in regulating many of the body's functions, including the stress response, blood pressure, and electrolyte balance. When the adrenal glands are not functioning properly, it can lead to a range of health issues, including fatigue, anxiety, and hormonal imbalances.

One way that Gua Sha can support adrenal health is by promoting relaxation and reducing stress. Chronic stress is one of the most common causes of adrenal fatigue, as it can lead to overproduction of cortisol and other stress hormones, which can eventually lead to burnout. By promoting relaxation and reducing stress, Gua Sha can help to support healthy adrenal function and prevent adrenal fatigue.

In addition to promoting relaxation, Gua Sha has also been found to have a direct effect on the adrenal glands themselves. A study published in the Journal of Acupuncture and Meridian Studies found that Gua Sha was effective at improving adrenal function in rats that had been exposed to chronic stress. The researchers found that Gua Sha helped to reduce cortisol levels and increase levels of other hormones that are important for adrenal function.

Another way that Gua Sha can support hormonal balance is by promoting healthy blood flow and circulation. Hormones are transported throughout the body via the bloodstream, and when circulation is compromised, it can lead to imbalances in hormone levels. Gua Sha has been found to improve circulation and increase blood flow to the areas where it is applied, which can help to promote healthy hormone levels.

1. Furthermore, Gua Sha has been found to have a balancing effect on the autonomic nervous system (ANS), which is responsible for regulating many of the body's functions, including hormone production. The ANS is made up of two branches: the sympathetic nervous system (SNS), which is responsible for the "fight or flight" response, and the parasympathetic nervous system (PNS), which is responsible for the "rest and digest" response. When the SNS is dominant, it can lead to overproduction of stress hormones and imbalances in the body. Gua Sha has been found to have a balancing effect on the ANS, helping to promote a more balanced state and healthy hormone levels.

## Gua Sha for Cardiovascular Health

Gua sha is an ancient healing technique that involves scraping the skin with a smooth-edged tool to stimulate blood flow, improve circulation, and promote healing. While it's often associated with musculoskeletal pain, gua sha can also be used to support cardiovascular health.

The cardiovascular system is responsible for delivering oxygen and nutrients to every cell in the body. When the cardiovascular system is compromised, it can lead to a host of health problems, including high blood pressure, heart disease, and stroke. Gua sha can help support cardiovascular health in several ways.

One way that gua sha can support cardiovascular health is by improving circulation. When the skin is scraped with a gua sha tool, it stimulates the production of nitric oxide, a molecule that helps dilate blood vessels and increase blood flow. This increased blood flow can help deliver oxygen and nutrients to the body's tissues more efficiently, which can improve overall cardiovascular function.

Another way that gua sha can support cardiovascular health is by reducing inflammation. Inflammation is a natural response to injury or infection, but when it becomes chronic, it can contribute to a variety of health problems, including cardiovascular disease. Gua sha can help reduce inflammation by stimulating the production of anti-inflammatory cytokines, which can help reduce inflammation throughout the body.

Gua sha can also help support cardiovascular health by reducing stress. Stress is a major contributor to cardiovascular disease, and chronic stress can cause long-term damage to the cardiovascular system. Gua sha can help reduce stress by promoting relaxation and reducing muscle tension, which can help lower blood pressure and support overall cardiovascular health.

Additionally, gua sha can help improve the health of the lymphatic system, which is closely linked to cardiovascular health. The lymphatic system is responsible for removing waste and toxins from the body, and when it becomes compromised, it can lead to inflammation and other health problems. Gua sha can help stimulate lymphatic drainage, which can help improve cardiovascular health by removing toxins and reducing inflammation.

When it comes to using gua sha for cardiovascular health, it's important to work with a qualified practitioner who can tailor the treatment to your specific needs. Gua sha is a powerful technique, and it's important to use it safely and effectively.

If you're interested in using gua sha to support your cardiovascular health, it's important to talk to your healthcare provider first. They can help you determine whether gua sha is a safe and appropriate treatment for your specific needs.

## Improving circulation

Gua sha is a traditional Chinese medicine technique that involves scraping the skin with a smooth-edged tool to promote healing and wellness. One of the many benefits of gua sha is its ability to improve circulation throughout the body. Below we will explore how gua sha can improve circulation, its benefits for overall health, and tips for incorporating gua sha into a daily routine.

Improved circulation is essential for maintaining good health. Blood carries oxygen and nutrients to all parts of the body, including the brain, heart, and muscles. When circulation is compromised, it can lead to a range of health problems, including heart disease, high blood pressure, and diabetes. Poor circulation can also cause symptoms such as numbness, tingling, and cold extremities.

Gua sha can help to improve circulation by breaking up stagnant blood and promoting the flow of fresh blood to the affected areas. The scraping motion of the gua sha tool creates small blood vessels, called capillaries, to dilate and increase blood flow to the skin and underlying tissues. This increased blood flow can help to flush out toxins and waste products, which can also improve overall health.

In addition to improving circulation, gua sha can provide numerous benefits for overall health. Regular gua sha can help to reduce inflammation and pain, boost the immune system, and relieve stress and anxiety. The technique can also improve the appearance of the skin, reducing fine lines and wrinkles and improving tone and texture.

To incorporate gua sha into a daily routine, it is essential to have the proper tools and technique. Gua sha tools come in a variety of shapes and sizes, including flat stones, spoons, and specially designed gua sha boards. The tool should be held at a 45-degree angle to the skin, with gentle pressure applied in a scraping motion. The skin should be lubricated with oil or lotion to prevent discomfort or irritation.

When using gua sha for circulation, it is essential to target the areas of the body with the most significant circulation issues. These areas may include the hands and feet, the scalp, or areas of the body affected by injury or chronic pain. Gua sha can be done daily, but it is important to avoid using too much pressure, as this can cause bruising or discomfort.

## Reducing blood pressure

Gua Sha is a traditional Chinese medicine technique that involves the use of a smooth-edged tool to scrape the skin. While it is most commonly used for musculoskeletal pain, it can also be effective in promoting cardiovascular health. Below we will explore the benefits of Gua Sha for reducing blood pressure and how it can be incorporated into a cardiovascular health regimen.

High blood pressure, or hypertension, is a major risk factor for cardiovascular disease. It is estimated that nearly half of all adults in the United States have high blood pressure. Hypertension can lead to serious health problems such as heart attacks, strokes, and kidney disease if left untreated. While medications are often prescribed to lower blood pressure, lifestyle changes such as regular exercise, a healthy diet, and stress reduction techniques can also be effective.

Gua Sha is a gentle and non-invasive technique that can be used in conjunction with other lifestyle changes to lower blood pressure. When the skin is scraped with a Gua Sha tool, it creates a mild trauma that triggers the body's natural healing response. This response increases blood flow to the area and can help reduce inflammation and promote healing.

One study published in the Journal of Traditional Chinese Medicine found that Gua Sha can lower blood pressure in patients with hypertension. The study involved 52 participants who were divided into two groups. One group received Gua Sha treatment twice a week for five weeks, while the other group received no treatment. The results showed that the group who received Gua Sha treatment had a significant decrease in both systolic and diastolic blood pressure compared to the control group.

Another study published in the Journal of Alternative and Complementary Medicine found that Gua Sha can improve blood circulation in patients with chronic obstructive pulmonary disease (COPD), a condition that often leads to pulmonary hypertension. The study involved 15 patients with COPD who received Gua Sha treatment once a week for four weeks. The results showed that Gua Sha improved blood circulation in the patients, which can help alleviate the symptoms of pulmonary hypertension.

In addition to its direct effects on blood pressure, Gua Sha can also be effective in reducing stress, which is another major risk factor for cardiovascular disease. When the body is under stress, it releases hormones such as cortisol and adrenaline, which can cause the heart to work harder and increase blood pressure. Gua Sha has been shown to reduce stress and promote relaxation, which can help lower blood pressure over time.

Incorporating Gua Sha into a cardiovascular health regimen can be done in several ways. One option is to see a licensed acupuncturist or Gua Sha practitioner who can perform the treatment. Another option is to purchase a Gua Sha tool and perform the treatment on oneself or a partner. It is important to note that proper technique and hygiene are essential to ensure the safety and effectiveness of the treatment.

Gua Sha can be performed on various parts of the body to promote cardiovascular health, including the neck, chest, back, and legs. It is important to start slowly and gradually increase the intensity of the treatment over time. The treatment should be performed for a few minutes at a time and repeated several times per week for best results.

## Gua Sha for Energy and Vitality

Gua Sha is a traditional Chinese healing technique that involves scraping the skin using a smooth-edged tool to stimulate circulation and promote healing. It has been used for thousands of years to treat a variety of health conditions and promote overall well-being, including boosting energy and vitality. Below we will explore the benefits of Gua Sha for energy and vitality, and how it works to promote these essential aspects of our health.

Gua Sha is believed to work by promoting the flow of qi, or vital energy, through the body's meridians, which are channels that connect different organs and tissues. When qi is blocked or stagnant, it can lead to various health problems, including fatigue and low energy levels. Gua Sha helps to remove these blockages and promote the free flow of qi, which can help to increase energy and vitality.

One of the primary benefits of Gua Sha for energy and vitality is that it helps to stimulate the lymphatic system, which is responsible for removing waste and toxins from the body. When the lymphatic system is functioning properly, it can help to boost the immune system and improve overall energy levels. Gua Sha helps to stimulate lymphatic drainage, which can help to remove toxins from the body and improve circulation.

Gua Sha also helps to improve blood circulation, which is essential for delivering oxygen and nutrients to the body's tissues and organs. When blood flow is sluggish, it can lead to fatigue and low energy levels. Gua Sha helps to increase blood circulation, which can help to improve energy and vitality.

Another way that Gua Sha promotes energy and vitality is by reducing inflammation in the body. Inflammation is a natural response to injury or infection, but when it becomes chronic, it can lead to various health problems, including fatigue and low energy levels. Gua Sha helps to reduce inflammation by promoting the release of cytokines, which are proteins that help to regulate the immune system and reduce inflammation.

In addition to promoting the flow of qi, improving lymphatic drainage, increasing blood circulation, and reducing inflammation, Gua Sha also helps to release tension and stress in the body. Stress is a major contributor to fatigue and low energy levels, and Gua Sha can help to relieve stress by promoting relaxation and reducing muscle tension.

There are several techniques that can be used to perform Gua Sha for energy and vitality. One popular technique is to use the tool to scrape along the spine and down the back, which can help to stimulate the nervous system and improve overall energy levels. Another technique is to scrape along the arms and legs, which can help to improve blood circulation and lymphatic drainage.

It is important to note that Gua Sha should be performed by a trained practitioner who understands how to use the tool safely and effectively. It should not be performed on areas of the body with broken skin, rashes, or other skin conditions, and it should not be performed on areas of the body that are inflamed or swollen.

In addition to Gua Sha, there are several other techniques that can be used to promote energy and vitality. These include acupuncture, massage, and herbal remedies. Acupuncture involves inserting thin needles into specific points on the body to promote the free flow of qi and improve energy levels. Massage involves manipulating the soft tissues of the body to promote relaxation and improve circulation. Herbal remedies can be used to help balance the body's energy and promote overall health and vitality.

## Boosting energy levels

Gua Sha is a traditional Chinese medicine practice that involves the use of a scraping tool to stimulate blood flow and promote healing in the body. While Gua Sha has been traditionally used for pain relief and relaxation, it can also be beneficial for boosting energy levels and promoting vitality.

There are many factors that can contribute to low energy levels, such as poor sleep, stress, and a lack of exercise. Gua Sha can be used in conjunction with other lifestyle changes to help boost energy levels and promote overall vitality.

One way that Gua Sha can help boost energy levels is by stimulating blood flow and increasing oxygenation to the body's tissues. This can help to improve overall circulation and promote a feeling of increased energy and vitality. Gua Sha can also help to release tension and reduce stress, which can contribute to feelings of fatigue and low energy levels.

Another way that Gua Sha can help boost energy levels is by promoting better sleep. Gua Sha can be used to help relax the body and calm the mind, which can promote better sleep and more restorative rest. When the body is well-rested, it is better able to function optimally and maintain higher energy levels throughout the day.

Gua Sha can also be used to help support the body's natural detoxification processes, which can help to promote overall health and vitality. When the body is able to efficiently eliminate toxins and waste products, it can function more efficiently and effectively, leading to increased energy levels and improved overall health.

In addition to these benefits, Gua Sha can also help to promote mental clarity and focus, which can further contribute to increased energy levels and overall vitality. By reducing stress and tension and promoting relaxation, Gua Sha can help to clear the mind and enhance mental clarity, which can lead to increased productivity and higher levels of energy throughout the day.

There are many different techniques and approaches that can be used with Gua Sha to help boost energy levels and promote overall vitality. Some practitioners may focus on specific acupressure points or meridians that are believed to be particularly effective for increasing energy and vitality, while others may use a more generalized approach to help promote overall relaxation and rejuvenation.

When incorporating Gua Sha into a wellness routine for boosting energy and vitality, it is important to work with a trained and experienced practitioner who can provide guidance and support throughout the process. Gua Sha should be used in conjunction with other lifestyle changes, such as getting enough sleep, eating a balanced and nutritious diet, and engaging in regular exercise, to promote optimal results.

## Cultivating life force energy (Qi)

Gua Sha, an ancient Chinese healing technique, has been used for centuries to promote wellness and balance in the body. One of the ways it achieves this is by promoting the flow of life force energy, also known as Qi (pronounced "chee"). Below we will explore how Gua Sha can be used to cultivate life force energy and promote overall vitality.

In traditional Chinese medicine, it is believed that Qi is the vital force that animates all living beings. When Qi is flowing freely, we feel energized, healthy, and balanced. However, when Qi becomes blocked or stagnant, we can experience a wide range of physical and emotional symptoms, such as fatigue, pain, and stress.

Gua Sha is a powerful tool for promoting the flow of Qi throughout the body. By using a Gua Sha tool to massage and scrape the skin, the technique can help release any tension or blockages in the muscles and connective tissue. As a result, Qi is able to flow more freely throughout the body, promoting a sense of vitality and balance.

There are several ways to use Gua Sha to cultivate life force energy. One of the most effective techniques is to focus on specific acupressure points along the body's meridian system. Meridians are channels through which Qi flows, and there are over 350 acupressure points along the body's meridians. By targeting specific points with Gua Sha, practitioners can help unblock any stagnant Qi and encourage the energy to flow freely.

Another way to use Gua Sha to cultivate Qi is to incorporate it into a daily self-care routine. Regular Gua Sha massage sessions can help release tension in the muscles and promote a sense of relaxation and wellbeing. By taking the time to care for our bodies and minds in this way, we can cultivate a deeper sense of connection to our life force energy and feel more energized and balanced throughout the day.

In addition to promoting the flow of Qi, Gua Sha can also help balance the body's yin and yang energies. Yin and yang are opposing forces that must be in balance for optimal health and vitality. When one energy is out of balance, it can manifest as physical or emotional symptoms. Gua Sha can help restore the balance of yin and yang energies by promoting the flow of Qi and releasing any tension or blockages in the body.

## Gua Sha for Spiritual Growth

Gua Sha is an ancient technique used in traditional Chinese medicine to treat various physical and emotional ailments. While it is commonly known for its ability to alleviate pain and tension in the body, Gua Sha can also be used as a tool for spiritual growth and self-discovery.

In traditional Chinese medicine, the body is viewed as a holistic system that is interconnected with the mind and spirit. According to this philosophy, physical and emotional health are closely linked, and it is believed that imbalances in the body can lead to disharmony in all areas of life. By using

Gua Sha to balance the body's energy and promote healing, individuals can experience not only physical benefits but also a deeper sense of spiritual connection and personal growth.

One of the primary ways that Gua Sha can support spiritual growth is by helping to release emotional blockages. When we experience negative emotions such as anger, grief, or fear, these feelings can become stuck in the body, leading to physical tension and discomfort. By using Gua Sha to stimulate the flow of Qi and blood in the body, these blockages can be released, allowing the individual to experience a greater sense of emotional freedom and clarity.

Gua Sha can also be used to support the development of mindfulness and self-awareness. During a Gua Sha session, the practitioner may encourage the individual to focus on their breath or to tune into the physical sensations in their body. By practicing mindfulness in this way, individuals can become more attuned to their inner experiences and develop a greater sense of self-awareness. This can lead to a deeper understanding of their own thoughts, feelings, and behaviors, and can support them in making positive changes in their lives.

Another way that Gua Sha can support spiritual growth is by promoting a sense of connection to the natural world. Traditional Chinese medicine views the body as a microcosm of the larger universe, with each part of the body corresponding to a different element or aspect of nature. By using Gua Sha to stimulate the flow of energy in the body, individuals can become more attuned to the natural rhythms of the world around them. This can promote a sense of connection to the earth, sky, and all living beings, leading to a deeper sense of spiritual connection and purpose.

In addition to its spiritual benefits, Gua Sha can also support physical health and well-being. By promoting the flow of Qi and blood in the body,

Gua Sha can help to reduce inflammation, improve circulation, and support the immune system. It can also be used to alleviate pain and tension in the muscles and joints, support digestion and respiratory function, and promote healthy skin.

To experience the spiritual benefits of Gua Sha, it is important to work with a qualified practitioner who is trained in this technique. During a Gua Sha session, the practitioner will use a smooth-edged tool to scrape the skin in a particular pattern, stimulating the flow of Qi and blood in the body. They may also use other traditional Chinese medicine techniques such as acupuncture, herbal medicine, or meditation to support the individual's overall health and well-being.

In addition to working with a practitioner, there are also practices that individuals can incorporate into their daily lives to support their spiritual growth. These may include mindfulness meditation, Qi Gong or Tai Chi, yoga, or other forms of physical exercise that promote the flow of energy in the body. It is also important to prioritize self-care practices such as getting enough sleep, eating a healthy diet, and taking time for relaxation and self-reflection.

## Connecting with your inner self

Gua Sha is an ancient Chinese healing technique that has been used for centuries to address a wide range of physical and emotional issues. While it is primarily known for its physical benefits, such as reducing pain and inflammation, it can also have a profound impact on one's spiritual growth and overall wellbeing.

At its core, Gua Sha is about creating balance and harmony within the body. This is accomplished by using a smooth, flat tool to apply pressure and friction to the skin, which helps to stimulate circulation, release tension, and activate the body's natural healing processes. As this process unfolds, it can have a profound impact on one's emotional and spiritual state as well.

One of the primary ways that Gua Sha can support spiritual growth is by helping individuals connect more deeply with their inner selves. This is because the physical sensations and movements of Gua Sha can help to bring awareness to the body and its needs, which in turn can help to cultivate a deeper sense of mindfulness and presence. By becoming more attuned to the body in this way, individuals can learn to listen more closely to their intuition and inner guidance, which can support them on their spiritual path.

In addition to helping individuals connect with their inner selves, Gua Sha can also support spiritual growth by promoting a sense of balance and harmony within the body. This is because many spiritual traditions teach that the body and mind are interconnected, and that imbalances or blockages in one can have a negative impact on the other. By using Gua Sha to release tension and promote circulation, individuals can create a more harmonious balance between their physical and emotional states, which can support them in cultivating a deeper sense of peace and wellbeing.

Another way that Gua Sha can support spiritual growth is by helping individuals release stored emotions and energetic blockages. Many of us carry emotional wounds or traumas that we may not even be aware of, and these can create blockages in our energy system that can affect our physical, emotional, and spiritual wellbeing. Gua Sha can help to release these blockages and bring these stored emotions to the surface, allowing individuals to process and release them in a healthy way. This can support individuals in releasing old patterns and beliefs that no longer serve them, and can open up space for new growth and transformation.

Finally, Gua Sha can support spiritual growth by helping individuals cultivate a deeper sense of self-love and acceptance. By using Gua Sha to nurture and care for the body, individuals can learn to treat themselves with more kindness and compassion, which can support them in developing a more positive and loving relationship with themselves. This can be a powerful step towards spiritual growth, as it can help individuals connect more deeply with their own innate worth and value.

## Enhancing mindfulness and meditation

Gua Sha is a traditional Chinese healing technique that involves scraping the skin with a flat tool to promote healing and relaxation. While commonly used for physical ailments, such as muscle tension and pain, Gua Sha can also be used to enhance mindfulness and meditation practices. Below we will explore how Gua Sha can help enhance mindfulness and meditation, and provide tips on how to incorporate this technique into your practice.

Mindfulness is a practice that involves being present and aware of the moment, without judgment or distraction. Meditation, on the other hand, is a practice that involves focusing the mind on a particular object or activity, to achieve a state of calm and relaxation. Both mindfulness and meditation have been shown to have numerous health benefits, including reducing stress and anxiety, improving sleep, and enhancing overall well-being.

Gua Sha can be a useful tool in enhancing these practices, as it helps to promote relaxation and reduce tension in the body. When the body is tense, it can be difficult to focus the mind and be present in the moment. By using Gua Sha to release tension and promote relaxation, it can be easier to enter a state of mindfulness or meditation.

One of the key benefits of Gua Sha is its ability to improve circulation and promote blood flow. When the body is tense, blood flow can become restricted, leading to a variety of health problems. By promoting circulation, Gua Sha helps to bring oxygen and nutrients to the cells, improving overall health and well-being. This improved circulation can also help to enhance the mind-body connection, making it easier to focus the mind and be present in the moment.

Another benefit of Gua Sha is its ability to release toxins from the body. When the body is full of toxins, it can be difficult to focus the mind and be present in the moment. By releasing these toxins, Gua Sha helps to promote a clear and focused mind, making it easier to enter a state of mindfulness or meditation.

Incorporating Gua Sha into your mindfulness or meditation practice can be easy and simple. Begin by finding a quiet and comfortable space where you can relax and focus on your breathing. Using a Gua Sha tool, gently scrape the skin in a downward motion, starting from the neck and working your way down the back. Repeat this process on the arms, legs, and other areas of the body as needed.

As you perform the Gua Sha technique, focus on your breath and the sensations in your body. Allow your mind to become present and aware of the moment, without judgment or distraction. If your mind begins to wander, gently bring your attention back to your breath and the sensations in your body.

In addition to using Gua Sha during mindfulness or meditation, it can also be used as a tool for self-care and relaxation. By incorporating Gua Sha into your daily routine, you can help to promote overall health and well-being, while also reducing stress and tension in the body.

To get the most out of your Gua Sha practice, it is important to use a high-quality Gua Sha tool and to follow proper technique. Be sure to apply gentle pressure and avoid using the tool on areas of the body that are sensitive or injured. If you have any concerns about using Gua Sha, be sure to consult with a healthcare provider before beginning.

## Gua Sha for Self-Care and Self-Love

Gua sha is an ancient Chinese practice that has gained popularity in recent years as a self-care technique. It involves using a tool, such as a smooth-edged stone or ceramic spoon, to scrape the skin gently in long strokes. Gua sha is often used in Traditional Chinese Medicine to alleviate pain and reduce inflammation, but it can also have benefits for self-care and self-love.

One way that gua sha can support self-care is by promoting relaxation and stress relief. As the tool is gently scraped over the skin, it can stimulate the body's natural healing processes and promote the flow of blood and energy. This can help to release tension and reduce feelings of anxiety or overwhelm. Gua sha can also be a soothing and calming self-care ritual, helping to promote feelings of self-love and self-nurturing.

Another benefit of gua sha for self-care is its ability to support skin health. The gentle scraping motion can help to improve circulation, which can promote a healthy, radiant complexion. Gua sha can also help to reduce puffiness and inflammation in the skin, particularly around the eyes, cheeks, and jawline. By incorporating gua sha into a regular self-care routine, individuals can promote healthy skin and enhance their overall sense of well-being.

In addition to its physical benefits, gua sha can also be a powerful tool for emotional self-care. The gentle, meditative nature of the practice can help individuals to connect with their inner selves and promote feelings of self-awareness and self-acceptance. By taking the time to slow down and engage in a mindful gua sha practice, individuals can cultivate a sense of inner peace and self-love.

To incorporate gua sha into a self-care routine, individuals can start by selecting a gua sha tool and learning the proper techniques for using it. There are many online resources and tutorials available that can guide beginners through the process. It's important to use a gentle touch and avoid applying too much pressure or scraping too hard. Gua sha should be a gentle and soothing practice, not a painful or uncomfortable one.

Once individuals have learned the basics of gua sha, they can begin to incorporate it into their regular self-care routine. This might involve setting aside time each day or week to engage in a gua sha practice, or incorporating it into a larger self-care routine that also includes other practices, such as meditation, yoga, or aromatherapy. By making gua sha a regular part of their self-care routine, individuals can support their overall physical, emotional, and spiritual well-being.

It's important to note that while gua sha can be a powerful tool for self-care and self-love, it is not a substitute for professional medical care or treatment. Individuals should always consult with a healthcare provider before beginning any new self-care or wellness practice, particularly if they have any underlying health conditions or concerns.

## Developing a self-care routine

Self-care has become an increasingly popular topic in recent years, as people recognize the importance of taking care of themselves both physically and mentally. Gua Sha, an ancient Chinese healing technique, is one practice that can be incorporated into a self-care routine. Gua Sha involves using a flat tool to apply pressure and friction to the skin, which can help improve circulation, release tension, and promote relaxation. Below we will explore the benefits of Gua Sha as a self-care practice and provide tips for developing a consistent routine.

One of the key benefits of Gua Sha is its ability to improve circulation. By stimulating the skin and underlying tissues, Gua Sha can increase blood flow and lymphatic drainage, helping to nourish cells and remove waste products from the body. This can have a number of positive effects, such as reducing inflammation, promoting tissue repair, and boosting overall immune function.

In addition to its physical benefits, Gua Sha can also help release tension and promote relaxation. By applying pressure and friction to the skin, Gua Sha can help relieve muscle tightness and reduce stress, leading to a sense of calm and well-being. This can be especially beneficial for those who struggle with anxiety or other stress-related conditions.

To incorporate Gua Sha into a self-care routine, it is important to start with the right tools and techniques. Gua Sha tools come in a variety of shapes and sizes, but typically feature a flat surface that can be used to apply pressure to the skin. Some common types of Gua Sha tools include jade rollers, gua sha boards, and rose quartz facial rollers. When choosing a tool, it is important to select one that feels comfortable and easy to use.

Once you have your Gua Sha tool, it is important to learn the proper technique. To begin, apply a small amount of oil or serum to your skin to help the tool glide smoothly. Next, hold the tool at a 45-degree angle and apply gentle pressure to the skin, moving in upward and outward strokes. It is important to avoid applying too much pressure or using a back-and-forth motion, as this can cause skin irritation or bruising.

When incorporating Gua Sha into a self-care routine, consistency is key. It is recommended to perform Gua Sha for a few minutes each day, either in the morning or evening. This can be a great way to start or end the day, helping to promote relaxation and prepare the body for rest.

In addition to using Gua Sha on the face, the technique can also be applied to other areas of the body, such as the neck, shoulders, and back. This can be especially beneficial for those who experience tension or pain in these areas, as Gua Sha can help relieve muscle tightness and improve circulation.

## Cultivating self-compassion

Self-compassion is a vital component of overall well-being, and it involves treating ourselves with kindness, understanding, and acceptance, just as we would a good friend. Self-compassion involves recognizing that we all make mistakes and suffer in life, and instead of criticizing ourselves for these imperfections, we should respond with kindness, understanding, and support.

Gua Sha is a traditional Chinese medicine practice that involves using a tool to scrape the skin gently. This practice is believed to have numerous physical and emotional benefits, including promoting relaxation, reducing stress, and improving circulation. Incorporating Gua Sha into a self-care routine can be an excellent way to cultivate self-compassion and promote overall well-being.

One way that Gua Sha can promote self-compassion is by encouraging individuals to take time for themselves. Gua Sha requires some time and attention, and it can be a peaceful and meditative experience. Engaging in this practice can remind individuals that it is essential to take time for themselves and prioritize self-care.

Gua Sha can also promote self-compassion by encouraging individuals to listen to their bodies. When using a Gua Sha tool, it is essential to pay attention to how the body is responding. If a particular area is painful or uncomfortable, it may be necessary to adjust the pressure or angle of the tool. This attention to the body can be an excellent reminder to listen to our bodies and respond to their needs, which is a key component of self-compassion.

Another way that Gua Sha can promote self-compassion is by reducing stress and promoting relaxation. When we are stressed, our bodies release hormones such as cortisol and adrenaline, which can lead to a variety of physical and emotional symptoms. By promoting relaxation and reducing stress, Gua Sha can help individuals feel calmer and more centered, which can increase their ability to practice self-compassion.

Additionally, Gua Sha can promote self-compassion by improving physical symptoms that may be causing distress. For example, if an individual is experiencing headaches or muscle tension, using a Gua Sha tool can help alleviate these symptoms. By reducing physical discomfort, individuals may be better able to focus on self-compassionate practices, such as positive self-talk or meditation.

It is important to note that while Gua Sha can be an excellent tool for promoting self-compassion, it should not be used as a replacement for professional mental health care. If an individual is struggling with mental health issues such as anxiety or depression, they should seek out professional support in addition to incorporating self-care practices such as Gua Sha into their routine.

Incorporating Gua Sha into a self-care routine can be an excellent way to cultivate self-compassion and promote overall well-being. This practice can encourage individuals to take time for themselves, listen to their bodies, reduce stress, and alleviate physical discomfort. By promoting these self-care practices, Gua Sha can help individuals cultivate self-compassion and develop a greater sense of overall well-being.

## Gua Sha Case Studies and Testimonials

Gua sha is a traditional Chinese medicine technique that involves using a smooth tool, often made of jade or rose quartz, to scrape the skin in a particular pattern. This technique has been used for thousands of years in China to improve health and treat various ailments. Today, it has gained popularity worldwide and has been used to alleviate pain, improve blood flow, and promote overall well-being. There are many case studies and testimonials that support the effectiveness of gua sha in treating different health issues.

One case study published in the Journal of Alternative and Complementary Medicine reported that a patient suffering from chronic neck pain for over a year experienced significant relief after receiving gua sha treatments. The patient underwent three sessions of gua sha, and after each session, their pain decreased by over 50%. By the end of the third session, the patient reported an 80% reduction in pain, and the relief lasted for several weeks.

Another case study published in the Journal of Acupuncture and Meridian Studies reported that a patient with frozen shoulder syndrome experienced complete pain relief and improved shoulder mobility after six gua sha sessions. The patient had been suffering from the condition for over a year and had tried other treatments without success. After the gua sha treatments, the patient's range of motion had significantly improved, and they were able to perform daily activities without pain.

In addition to pain relief, gua sha has also been found to be effective in treating skin conditions. A case study published in the Journal of Traditional Chinese Medicine reported that a patient with severe acne experienced significant improvement in their skin after undergoing gua sha treatments. The patient received gua sha on their face twice a week for four weeks, and by the end of the treatment, their acne had reduced by 50%, and their skin tone and texture had improved.

Furthermore, gua sha has been found to be effective in treating chronic conditions such as fibromyalgia. A case study published in the Journal of Pain Research reported that a patient with fibromyalgia experienced significant pain relief after receiving gua sha treatments. The patient underwent ten sessions of gua sha, and by the end of the treatment, their pain levels had decreased by 50%, and their quality of life had significantly improved.

There are also many testimonials from people who have experienced the benefits of gua sha. One person reported that after receiving gua sha treatments for their migraines, they had not experienced a migraine for over six months. Another person reported that after receiving gua sha treatments for their anxiety, they felt calmer and more relaxed, and their anxiety symptoms had significantly reduced.

Gua sha has also been found to be effective in improving athletic performance. A study published in the Journal of Traditional Chinese Medicine reported that gua sha increased grip strength and reduced muscle soreness in athletes. The athletes received gua sha treatments on their forearms, and by the end of the treatment, their grip strength had increased by 7.5% and their muscle soreness had significantly decreased.

## Real-life experiences

Real-life experiences are powerful tools for understanding the impact of certain practices and techniques. When it comes to Gua Sha, there are many individuals who have experienced its benefits firsthand. From alleviating pain to promoting relaxation and improving skin health, Gua Sha has been shown to have a wide range of benefits. Below we will explore some real-life experiences of individuals who have incorporated Gua Sha into their self-care routine and have seen positive results.

One individual, Sarah, had been struggling with chronic neck and shoulder pain for years. Despite trying various therapies and medications, the pain persisted. She was introduced to Gua Sha by a friend and decided to give it a try. After a few sessions, she noticed a significant reduction in her pain and tension. She continued to receive Gua Sha treatments regularly and has found that her pain has subsided and her mobility has improved.

Another individual, John, had been experiencing stress and anxiety due to his demanding job. He had tried various relaxation techniques, but had not found anything that was effective for him. He came across Gua Sha and decided to give it a try. He found that the technique helped him to relax and let go of tension in his body. He now incorporates Gua Sha into his weekly self-care routine and has found that it has had a positive impact on his overall mental and emotional wellbeing.

For individuals struggling with skin issues, Gua Sha has also been shown to be beneficial. One woman, Emily, had been dealing with acne for years and had tried numerous treatments with little success. She was introduced to Gua Sha by a skincare professional and decided to incorporate it into her routine. She found that regular Gua Sha treatments helped to reduce inflammation and improve circulation, which in turn helped to improve the appearance of her skin. She now uses Gua Sha regularly as a part of her skincare routine and has found that her skin is much clearer and healthier.

Gua Sha has also been shown to be effective for individuals dealing with digestive issues. One man, Tom, had been struggling with acid reflux and indigestion for years. He had tried various medications and dietary changes with little success. He decided to try Gua Sha and found that it helped to promote better digestion and reduce his symptoms. He now receives regular Gua Sha treatments and has found that his digestive issues have significantly improved.

For individuals looking to improve their overall health and wellbeing, Gua Sha has also been shown to be beneficial. One woman, Maria, had been feeling generally unwell and fatigued. She had tried various supplements and diets, but had not found anything that helped. She decided to try Gua Sha and found that it helped to promote better circulation and energy flow throughout her body. She now uses Gua Sha regularly as a part of her self-care routine and has found that she has more energy and feels much better overall.

These real-life experiences demonstrate the potential benefits of Gua Sha for a wide range of issues. While it is important to note that every individual's experience may differ, these examples highlight the versatility and effectiveness of this technique. Whether you are dealing with pain, stress, skin issues, digestive problems, or simply looking to improve your overall health and wellbeing, Gua Sha may be worth exploring.

## Tips and advice from Gua Sha practitioners

Gua Sha, a traditional Chinese therapy technique, has gained popularity in recent years for its various health benefits, including reducing muscle tension, improving circulation, and promoting overall well-being. As more people turn to Gua Sha for its therapeutic effects, it's important to receive advice and tips from experienced practitioners to ensure proper technique and maximize the benefits of this practice. Below we will we'll discuss tips and advice from Gua Sha practitioners to help you get the most out of your Gua Sha experience.

1. Tip #1: Choose the Right Tool

The first and most important tip when starting Gua Sha is to choose the right tool. While there are many types of Gua Sha tools available in the market, such as jade, rose quartz, and stainless steel, it's essential to find one that suits your skin type and your level of experience. For beginners, a simple tool made of soft material such as jade or rose quartz is recommended. For more experienced users, a stainless steel tool can provide a more intense and deeper massage.

2. Tip #2: Apply Proper Pressure

When using Gua Sha, it's crucial to apply the right amount of pressure to avoid causing damage to the skin. According to Gua Sha practitioners, the amount of pressure you use should be enough to produce a mild discomfort but not so much that it causes pain or leaves bruises. The goal is to promote blood flow and improve circulation, not to cause harm.

3. Tip #3: Use Proper Technique

Proper technique is key to achieving the full benefits of Gua Sha. According to practitioners, the technique involves using short, firm strokes on the skin, always moving in an upward motion. The strokes should be done slowly and deliberately, starting from the center of the face or body and moving outwards. It's essential to avoid making back-and-forth movements or applying too much pressure in one area, as this can lead to skin damage.

4. Tip #4: Use the Right Products

To enhance the benefits of Gua Sha, it's recommended to use the right skincare products before and after the massage. Before Gua Sha, it's best to use a facial oil or serum to provide lubrication and allow the tool to glide smoothly over the skin. After the massage, a moisturizer can help to lock in the benefits of the massage and keep the skin hydrated.

5. Tip #5: Make it a Regular Practice

Like any other form of therapy or self-care, consistency is key to seeing results with Gua Sha. While a single session can provide temporary relief, incorporating Gua Sha into your regular routine can lead to long-lasting benefits such as improved skin texture, reduced muscle tension, and increased relaxation. It's recommended to perform Gua Sha 2-3 times per week for best results.

Testimonials

Gua Sha has been praised by many for its various benefits. Below are a few testimonials from individuals who have experienced the benefits of Gua Sha firsthand.

"I suffer from chronic neck and shoulder pain, and Gua Sha has been a lifesaver. Not only has it helped to relieve tension in my muscles, but it's also improved the texture of my skin and reduced the appearance of fine lines." - Jane, 42

"After incorporating Gua Sha into my skincare routine, I've noticed a significant improvement in the overall health of my skin. It looks brighter, smoother, and more even-toned." - Sarah, 29

"I've struggled with insomnia for years, but since starting Gua Sha, I've been able to fall asleep more easily and stay asleep longer. It's been a game-changer for my sleep and overall well-being." - Tom, 37

## Gua Sha Resources and Continuing Education

Gua Sha is an ancient healing technique that has been used in traditional Chinese medicine for centuries. It involves using a tool to scrape the skin in a specific pattern, which is believed to release tension, promote circulation, and alleviate pain. While Gua Sha is a simple technique, there are many different tools and approaches that practitioners use to achieve different effects.

If you're interested in learning more about Gua Sha or becoming a practitioner yourself, there are many resources and continuing education opportunities available to you. Below we will we'll explore some of these resources and how they can help you expand your knowledge and skills.

One great resource for learning about Gua Sha is books. There are many books available on the topic, ranging from introductory guides to advanced techniques. Some of the most popular books on Gua Sha include "The Complete Guide to Modern Gua Sha Therapy" by Clive Witham, "The Healing Power of Gua Sha" by Arya Nielsen, and "The Great Gua Sha Handbook" by Dr. Xu Xiangcai. These books provide detailed instructions and illustrations for various Gua Sha techniques, as well as information on the history and theory behind the practice.

In addition to books, there are also many online resources available for learning about Gua Sha. Many practitioners offer online courses and workshops that cover various aspects of Gua Sha, from basic techniques to advanced approaches. Some of these courses are self-paced, allowing you to learn at your own pace, while others are live and interactive, providing an opportunity to ask questions and interact with other students.

Another great way to learn about Gua Sha is through continuing education programs. Many massage therapy and acupuncture schools offer courses on Gua Sha, as well as other traditional Chinese medicine techniques. These programs are typically more comprehensive than online courses or workshops, providing a deeper understanding of the underlying theory and principles of Gua Sha. They also often include hands-on training, allowing you to practice your skills under the guidance of an experienced practitioner.

If you're already a practitioner of Gua Sha, there are also many continuing education opportunities available to help you expand your skills and knowledge. One option is to attend advanced workshops or conferences that focus on specific aspects of Gua Sha, such as facial Gua Sha or Gua Sha for fertility. These events often feature expert speakers and hands-on training, providing an opportunity to learn new techniques and network with other practitioners.

Another way to continue your education in Gua Sha is to seek out mentorship from experienced practitioners. This can be done through formal mentorship programs or by reaching out to practitioners in your area and asking to observe or assist in their sessions. By learning from experienced practitioners, you can gain valuable insights into their techniques and approaches, as well as receive feedback on your own skills.

In addition to formal resources and continuing education programs, it's also important to seek out opportunities to practice and refine your Gua Sha skills. This can be done by volunteering at local health clinics or offering Gua Sha sessions to friends and family. By practicing regularly, you can build your confidence and improve your technique, while also helping others experience the many benefits of Gua Sha.

## Staying updated on new techniques and research

Gua Sha, a traditional Chinese therapy that involves scraping the skin with a smooth tool, has gained popularity in recent years for its various health benefits. As more and more people become interested in this practice, new techniques and research are constantly emerging. It's important for practitioners and individuals to stay updated on these developments to ensure they are getting the most out of their Gua Sha practice. Below we will explore the importance of staying updated on new Gua Sha techniques and research, and provide some tips for doing so.

Firstly, it's important to understand the potential benefits of staying updated on new Gua Sha techniques and research. By doing so, practitioners and individuals can enhance the effectiveness of their practice and stay informed on any new findings or developments. For example, recent studies have shown that Gua Sha can help reduce inflammation, promote relaxation, and improve overall well-being. Staying up-to-date on these findings can help individuals understand how to use Gua Sha to target specific health issues.

In addition to staying informed on the potential benefits of Gua Sha, keeping up with new techniques can also improve the overall experience of the practice. New tools, methods, and techniques are constantly being developed that can make Gua Sha more comfortable, effective, and enjoyable. For example, some practitioners have begun incorporating aromatherapy into their Gua Sha practice, using essential oils to enhance relaxation and promote healing. By staying updated on these new techniques, individuals can make their Gua Sha practice more tailored and personalized to their specific needs.

So, how can practitioners and individuals stay updated on new Gua Sha techniques and research? Here are some tips:

1. Attend workshops and conferences: One of the best ways to stay updated on new Gua Sha techniques and research is to attend workshops and conferences. These events provide an opportunity to learn from experi-

enced practitioners and researchers, as well as network with others in the field.

2. Read books and articles: There are many books and articles available on Gua Sha, ranging from beginner's guides to in-depth studies on the topic. By reading these resources, individuals can stay informed on new techniques and research.

3. Follow experts on social media: Many Gua Sha practitioners and researchers have a social media presence, where they share their expertise and insights. By following these individuals on platforms such as Instagram and Twitter, individuals can stay updated on new developments in the field.

4. Join online communities: There are many online communities dedicated to Gua Sha, where practitioners and individuals can share their experiences, ask questions, and learn from others. By joining these communities, individuals can stay connected with others in the field and stay informed on new techniques and research.

5. Take continuing education courses: Many organizations offer continuing education courses on Gua Sha, which can help practitioners stay updated on new techniques and research. These courses can also help individuals develop their skills and knowledge in the field.

SD - #0152 - 070926 - C0 - 229/152/12 - PB - 9781776968244 - Matt Lamination